# Living With Chronic Pain

## From Ok To Despair And Finding My Way Back Again

Dr Dawn Macintyre

16pt

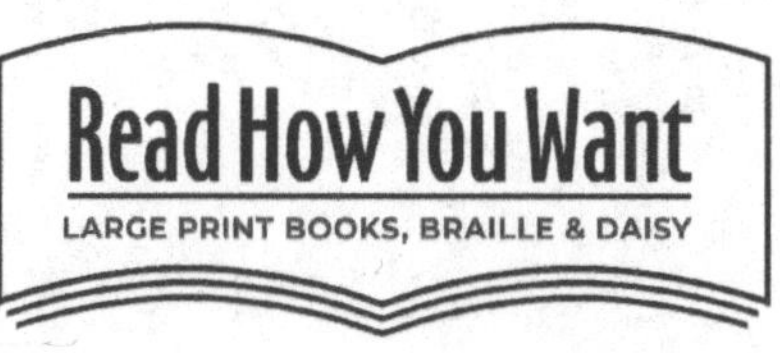

# Copyright Page from the Original Book



First published 2020



Big Sky Publishing Pty Ltd
PO Box 303, Newport, NSW 2106, Australia
Phone: 1300 364 611
Fax: (61 2) 9918 2396
Email: info@bigskypublishing.com.au
Web: www.bigskypublishing.com.au

Cover design and typesetting: Think Productions
Printed in China by Jilin GIGO International

A catalogue record for this book is available from the National Library of Australia

## TABLE OF CONTENTS

*This book is dedicated to all of us unwilling members of the pain tribe who fight every day to be the best we can be.*

# FOREWORD

It gives me great pleasure to be invited to endorse *Living with Chronic Pain, From OK to Despair and Finding My Way Back Again.* I have been aware Dawn was writing this book for several years and have been looking forward to the day I could read it. I was captivated from page one. Dawn drew me in with her easy conversational style. She also brings a unique perspective to the literature on pain as she has the experience from both sides of the health care system. That is, she has serious and complex health conditions which cause her chronic pain and secondly, she has worked as a health professional for more than thirty years.

When I founded the Australian Pain Management Association in 2009 my mantra to myself (it kept me sane) and other patients was: 'Your pain is real and there is a physical cause. You are not making it up!' The big change came for me when I learnt that it 'wasn't all in my head' but my brain was/is sending the pain through the network of nerves to my leg and foot even though these are numb but otherwise basically fine. My focus changed from wanting it fixed to: 'I can band together the skills and habits that work for me and keep at it every day.' My pain is now five or below (out of ten).

This book explores the critical issue of chronic pain which affects more than 3.4 million of us in Australia. Back pain is the leading cause of disability both here and globally. Ongoing pain causes enormous suffering for the patient but also for their family and friends. It is common for Australians living with chronic pain to develop depression and they are twice as likely to take their own lives. Dawn was not immune to the ravages of chronic pain 'when the pain took charge'. Medication didn't work at all, every movement was beyond endurance, she was unable to talk to loved ones and panic stricken that the doctors had no more tricks left. Reading Dawn's raw account of her worst agony and indignity vividly demonstrates the depths of the physical and mental anguish of chronic pain. At this nadir, when Dawn was most frustrated by the usual hospital clinicians, it was a hospital physiotherapist who listened to what she really needed and that encounter commenced Dawn's very gradual and ongoing rehabilitation.

Dawn's story may well become your survival guide. Alongside her personal story of pain also sits the narrative of self-care. There are not enough specialised pain clinics to help everyone with chronic pain so self-help is critically important and can lessen the slide into distress and incapacity. In this book, Dawn's journey illustrates how self-help can be effective and empowering when it is combined with the strategies given at health appointments. Dawn learns to walk beside her treating health professionals, working in partnership rather than expecting them to come up with the answers. As she says, 'I got control of my pain.' That's empowering for all of us!

You can have a lot of pain even when the body has healed. This is often a hard concept for patients to understand and accept ... it was for me.

However, gaining a sense of pain as a complex 'thing' can lead to the evidence-based therapies making more sense. This book presents the central elements of Acceptance and Commitment Theory and Cognitive Behaviour Therapy amongst others in a bright and engaging way. Discovering that thinking affects moods, and both affect pain can be an important part of the plan leading to managing the worst aspects of pain.

This book is also for health professionals working with people with chronic pain. If you want great insight into living with pain from an author who also speaks health care language and believes in evidence-based medicine, then this book is for you. This book goes a long way to improving understanding of people who live with pain and the stigma we face.

Finally, if you are a loved one, friend or colleague of someone who lives with the unpredictability of chronic pain, Appendix 1: *Behind the Mask: Conversations and Interviews* is for you. In this chapter, Dawn's foster daughter, Shae, a nurse, gives her account about watching her mother in agony and feeling feeble and unable to help. In my opinion, she helped a great deal as being there really helps. This is one of several fascinating interviews and windows into how pain affects these brave and persevering individuals.

Your pain is real and there is a physical cause. You are not making it up!

I am sure you will get much assistance and insight from this book.

Elizabeth Carrigan
Chief Executive Officer
Australian Pain Management Association

# TESTIMONIALS

*Living with Chronic Pain, From OK to Despair and Back Again* is a compelling autobiographical account of life with chronic pain, that will be invaluable to a wide audience. Written by a clinical counsellor from the interface of her personal experiences and professional background, it articulates the need for professionals to address the whole person, not just the parts, and understand the many-faceted enemy that pain can be for chronic sufferers. Equally, it role-models for pain sufferers, the mental strategies and self-reflection process that make what can be overwhelming, ultimately manageable. And last but not least, of course, sufferers who find it hard to get out the words that will help those around them understand might want to share their copy with (or buy one for) friends and family, as it speaks the common language of 'the pain tribe' of which Dawn, like all sufferers, are 'unwilling members.' I can see my pain clients in every line.

**Dr. Travis Gee, Psychologist, Pain Specialists Australia, Melbourne**

As a physiotherapist, I feel anxious when I go and see people with chronic pain. I know what I am going to say and how well I say it can be difficult. I know translating new knowledge without inquiring into a person's experience of what and how living with chronic pain is fraught. When I can drop this agenda and allow time to talk about their experience we can get somewhere. Dawn's book, by making this process so clear, gives me and other practitioners permission to step outside our dogma and prescribed roles to join together for a different experience to emerge. These safe conversations are only possible due to Dawn's generosity and courage and how she enables her experiences to be felt, shared and understood. It is only through this new understanding of how it is to live with chronic pain that we can continue to work in what is often a complex and intense human experience for both practitioner and the person with chronic pain.

**Sharon Barlow, Physiotherapist**

Despite Dawn and I having different 'causality' to our spinal and chronic pain, we share many similarities as women, mothers and partners. This raw, honest and refreshing personal account of both chronic pain and the harrowing impact to life – attempting to maintain a career and humanity is undeniably pivotal in the acceptance of chronic pain and finding a life thereafter.

**Sumarah, Chronic pain survivor**

Finally, a raw, authentic book that shares the real challenges of living with chronic pain. Dawn's insights into how her life was challenged, how stigma and guilt became all-consuming, and how she has turned it round to help both professionals and those living with chronic pain to identify what they need from family, friends and health professionals, makes this book the bible for everyone who knows or works with people living with chronic pain.

**Jan Sky, Neuropsychotherapist, Clinical Hypnotherapist and developer of ESI Mapping**

I believe this book fills a valuable part of the puzzle about the relationship between chronic pain and depression. What Dawn has done with her experience is provide validation for others who are going through the same or similar illness. It lets them know they are not alone. I would like Dawn to speak at insurance industry conferences, so advisors and agents have a better understanding of the support needs of their clients.

**Ben Wilshire,**
**Lion and Shield Insurance and Financial Services**

- Thrive and survive with this wonderful chronic pain chronicle.
- Smile in recognition, and cry with this book, but most of all, learn about chronic pain and the way out of suffering.
- Enter the shadows of chronic pain and then emerge into the light that you will be able to switch on yourself.
- This book is a clear window into chronic pain and the image is

sharp. Contemplate too, the bright horizon.

- Take this surprising voyage of chronic pain; into your work in the clinic or into your life as a patient.

**Elizabeth Carrigan, Chief Executive Officer, Australian Pain Management Association Limited (APMA)**

# INTRODUCTION

## ***It's all in your head—they said!***

Welcome to sharing my thoughts and experiences of love, life and chronic pain. And while this is definitely my story, I know that there are many parts of my journey that will resonate, because sadly, chronic pain is now in epidemic proportions. One in five of us experience chronic pain in our lives and after 60 years of age that figure goes to one in three. So, you are likely reading this either because you have to live with chronic pain, or you know someone who does.

I originally titled this book *When Everything Changes—Walk with Me* because since my first book *Nothing Changes if Nothing Changes* was published in 2008, there have been numerous changes in my life – both personally and professionally. But I wasn't sure you would pick the book up with that title. I was concerned it wouldn't hit you between the eyes enough and make clear exactly what I wanted to share with you in this story. But I hope you do walk alongside me as you read this, as I hope to walk alongside you, sharing my experiences, those of a few other chronic pain sufferers (or do I say 'survivors'?) and maybe even reflecting the experiences of you, or someone your love, who is living with chronic pain. Importantly, my motivation behind writing this book is to share experiences that are not often discussed, a bit like the elephant in the room. I don't want to talk about the medical side of pain – my story is about the social and psychological impact, specifically non-specific or nondisease related chronic pain. I share with you the changes in my life as chronic pain became the dominant factor; as chronic pain invaded my body over the years, the changes I had to make, the changes I chose to make and my final acceptance that I have, and can live with chronic pain.

I have always been a believer in 'mind over matter'; if we are mentally focussed and positive, so much can be achieved. I know that some people are more motivated than others, maybe due to personality differences, maybe life circumstances, or perhaps a combination of both – you know, the nature/nurture argument. I happen to be born with a subtle determination to succeed even though I don't think I was conscious of this until my early 20's. I have been branded as having an 'A' type personality (ambitious, organised and perhaps a little impatient). Maybe some of us are just naturally more positive in attitude and outlook than others – the glass half-empty, half-full scenario.

Yet in 2013, half-full seemed an exaggeration and a mockery of my life. My back pain was constant and exhausting, possibly an accumulation of multiple surgeries over my lifetime, and a riding accident when I was 14 years old. I struggled to find even a drop of joy, let alone a puddle to grace the bottom of a glass. Recurring bouts of pain left me desperate and exhausted, in what was to become the beginning of a new chapter in my life, a chapter that told a story, my story of flare-ups, brain fog, fear, distraction, absorption, isolation, exhaustion, constant pain that never left me day or night, and on a frustrating medical merry-go-round in a desperate bid to find answers. Inevitable fights with Google and all the legitimate and less favourable research out there only served to confuse me even more.

And suddenly – no, not suddenly, in fact it was a slow insidious build-up that was wearing me down until I finally reached my tipping (or should I say, crashing) point, I didn't have one positive thought in any cell of my body. I knew I didn't want to continue my life this way. I felt a total burden, a waste of space, a thief of quality air that others were better able to utilise. And the biggest, calmest thought was that I wanted to kill myself. That was a much easier and bearable option than the current recurring situation. I wasn't being dramatic or attention-seeking. Actually, quite the opposite. I was fed up with the attention which was no longer about the fun-filled Dawn, the intelligent Dawn, the animal-loving Dawn, the caring Dawn or the interesting person. No, all the attention from myself and (I believed) others was based on my pain, my inability to socialise anymore, and my complete loss of confidence in my world as I knew it.

I felt a burden to my husband and my children, and it wasn't safe to be around the grandchildren for fear that they would get freaked out by the intensity of my pain. Entertaining the idea of travelling to see my family in the UK became a total farce. The only non-judgemental aspect of my life was being with my gorgeous dogs, despite their walks being significantly curtailed. Not the same for our four lovely goats however, who got the raw end of the deal. As my ability to look after them became erratic and unreliable, we sadly had to rehome them. So why couldn't I adopt my life-learned approach of thinking positively and resolving the issue? I was exhausted. Exhausted from constant pain, exhausted from no more answers and as each day offered no way out or what I considered a quality way to cope with the pain, I truly had nothing left to draw upon.

My pain isn't related to a specific disease like cancer, so it was more difficult to understand the 'why'. I refer to this as nondisease-related chronic pain (NDRCP), a phrase which probably applies to many sufferers in Australia. I have also heard this referred to as non-specific chronic pain so I am assuming these terms are interchangeable. I was also on significant amounts of medication which meant I wasn't able to think clearly – or was it the pain causing that? One of the medications was for neuropathic pain, but also an antidepressant. Even with that supposed chemical support, nothing was changing. I had had all the surgery I was prepared to undergo, attended pain clinics and pain-management programs, drawn upon my knowledge of cognitive behaviour therapy, lifestyle changes, nutrition and sleep hygiene, exercise etc. and I was still in the same place!

And so this book. Whilst there is acknowledgement for the need to address NDRCP in a multidisciplinary fashion, in my experience little seems to be available regarding ongoing support. You see, the very nature of NDRCP means it's not going away soon – if ever. We exhaust every known avenue of doctors, medication, chronic pain specialists, rehabilitation, pain clinics, pain programs, physiotherapists, psychologists, naturopathy, homeopathy, Pilates, swimming, acupuncture, diversion therapy – the list goes on, and so for many of us does the pain.

So what would be useful to those of us for whom NDRCP is going to be as much a part of our lives as the air we breathe and the ground that we walk on? What is the support gap that needs filling to help live a worthwhile life again?

In order to answer this question, it is important to understand many of the elements that NDRCP affects in our lives. I realised that living with NDRCP is similar to living with constant grief and loss, the subject of my doctoral thesis some years ago. We have to learn to adapt to 'the new normal' and each of us will do this in different ways. One thing is for sure, leaving us unsupported to cope after we have been through some, or all, of the above efforts to resolve our pain has the potential to actually create more negative and depressing thoughts and behaviours. After all, if we have tried everything we could find and still feel like this – what hope is there?

This is where I can come in.

Sharing my lived experience, my professional expertise as a clinical counsellor with a clinical and academic interest in loss and grief, I hope my story will resonate with those with chronic pain: the sufferer, and those living with the one suffering. I have written this book from the heart in the hope that my story, my voice, helps other chronic pain sufferers, and so their families and friends also have their voices heard. I hope that through my journey I can help validate and authenticate the challenges and discoveries that we reluctant members of this unwanted pain tribe experience.

Intentionally, this book is NOT a 'how-to' guide. There are a few good books already available in that genre, but when I was in agony, exhausted and feeling so alone, those books seemed to be referring to 'the others', not me. However, I have provided a list of reflections at the end of each chapter, some insights into what I have learnt and what you can possibly do to alleviate your journey as a sufferer or someone who lives or works with a person in chronic pain.

On reflection, part of that difficulty I had early on in dealing with my chronic pain was that I was asking the wrong questions, using the wrong words. I was desperate for someone to find an answer to my situation. Instead, I needed to look for a way to manage my condition and my life that had been so critically impacted by the constant pain. I had to have my condition validated, to be believed, to hold my head up high and find hope again.

This book is not an academic exercise, nor does it intend to explain pain in great detail. This is my account of joyous times, desperate times and discovery. My life is once again rich and full of opportunity, though not void of the unpredictable, the fear and frustration of the inevitable flare-ups and invasion into my physical and emotional space. I hope that by telling my story you will gain some insight into how NDRCP affects many of us, and that you and your families can have a greater understanding and more open conversations about this life-changing condition and how we can support each other.

Making sense of pain is a godsend. It's the beginning of believing in a better future.

But let me start at the beginning...

# Part One

# The Beginning

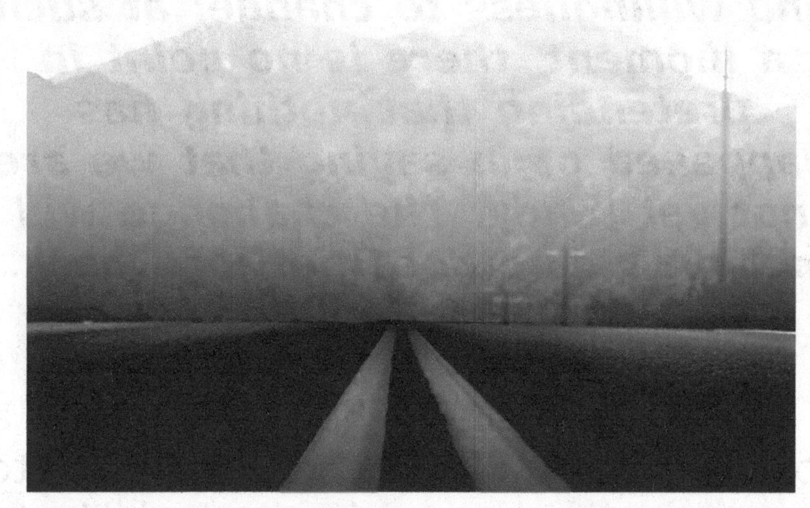

# 1

# MY ROAD MAP

***When we least expect it, life sets us a challenge to test our courage and willingness to change; at such a moment, there is no point in pretending that nothing has happened or in saying that we are not yet ready. The challenge will not wait. Life does not look back.***
**Paulo Coelho**

I never realised how important a road map could be, especially to someone who has an innate inability to read maps and is forever grateful to live in a world where technology has provided us with a GPS. My road map has been both my lifesaver and my life challenger. My GPS hasn't always sent me on the correct route. It bears the name 'my flower'. Meet my stomach scar, a much more delicate and gentle vision than the harshness and confusion of a map, especially as flowers make me smile, bring me light, joy and happiness. Maps cause me confusion and anxiety, get me lost and feeling inadequate, confused, and like I'm going around and around in circles.

I carry it with me every day, have done since I was ten days old and it has grown bigger and more complex with each year of my life. I wear it as a badge of life, not a badge of honour but a mark of my inevitability, my unique passage through a world of challenges and pain. In the days of midriffs and bikinis, I was never able to dress like my friends, my flower being a drawcard for eye focus, and then aversion. It's a complex course, less clear than the Monopoly board taking you through the streets of London, or the Tube map guiding you through and across its complex rail and tunnel systems. No, my own personal map is one that got me lost every time, most years offering yet a new direction, new links and connections to its platform – platforms that I didn't choose to wait on. One thing was reliable though: whilst I would often get lost trying to navigate my way around the many twists and turns now tattooed on my stomach, I would always end up at the central point, that being me, the confused, messy cluster in the middle from where most roads led and all returned.

When my two daughters reached the age of enquiry, that beautiful innocent wonder when they realised not all things were the same, rather than becoming critics, they were still at the stage of acceptance, of seeing things for what they were, without judgement. Of course, they only ever knew me with my scars. One day Taryn and Kara asked why my tummy was different to theirs, and why I didn't have a belly button like they did. The road map analogy seemed a little out of their ken, so I told them I was so lucky. I have this flower that is always with me, that makes me smile and is my lifeline. My flower needs to be loved and cared for every day, watered in the shower; by looking after it, my life and its life are totally intertwined, connected by a life force that is mine and mine alone. How lucky was I to carry something with me at all times, something so beautiful and special. I told them we all have our own unique beauty, something that we have to look after ourselves and then it in turn will look after us. For some, it's a physical thing that everyone can see, for others it's something deep inside, something connected to their heart and soul. That seemed to satisfy them for the time being and my road map became lovingly known as 'my flower' from that day forth.

But flowers don't bloom and sustain themselves all year round. Mine was no different. It saw many a challenging season, a time when it struggled to survive and needed new input, new fertiliser to stay alive in this harsh world. My flower has seen 16 seasons of change, 16 different surgeries creating new directions in both a physical and psychological direction. It was only in my mid-50's that I realised how this flower, the seasons, the confusing road map, has affected my life. It's only now that I understand how, with so much of my stomach removed, sewn up, connected and reconnected, my back pain is intrinsically connected to these imposts. After all, how can my back hold itself strong and upright when all my core muscles have been ravaged since day ten of their very existence! My neural pathways were compromised from very early on. The connection seems so obvious now that I have learnt so much about chronic pain. But these connections were never made for me over all the years. Link that with my accident when I was 14 years old, and yes, my pain makes perfect sense.

## Reflections from this Chapter

- Chronic pain is often a learned experience resulting in learned behaviours. This also means that there is an opportunity to unlearn behaviours and discover new ones.
- Recognising that we are unique, with our own journey to navigate, is a key to being in control.
- The brain can default and once we know this, we can learn how to set it back on the right pathway.
- Do you understand the connection between past experiences and your chronic pain? Reflecting on this is

a good start to finding a way forward.

# 2

# MY FIRST 20 YEARS

***It is not in the stars to hold our destiny but in ourselves.***
**William Shakespeare**

I believe my destiny was rubber stamped on 19 January 1959, ten days after I was born. My parents named me Dawn, and it's only in recent years that I have come to appreciate the meaning of my first name; the beginning of a new day, hope, fresh starts, new possibilities. There were times when I thought it was given to me as some sort of joke, a way of mocking my very existence, the fact that I had to keep facing another day, another round of desperate agony.

My entry into the world was perfect – full of joy and happiness for my parents, completing their family of three children. However, ten days later I developed a bowel blockage and required emergency surgery. This set a pattern in motion, a destiny that was to be my path through life and shape the person I am today. I had the first of multiple surgeries over my lifetime, with a bowel resection and a colostomy bag for the first three months of my little life. What a disruption for my family: Mum's otherwise perfect life was suddenly thrown into upheaval. Although she was fortunate enough to have au pairs, home help and close family support, she still had the emotional anguish of her newborn daughter being so unwell, in hospital for three months and having to be a mum for my siblings, Lorraine and Gary, who were only fifteen months old and four at the time. Not exactly the picture of maternal bliss she had in mind.

As a child, I enjoyed the love of both my parents and the security of a comfortable and happy home, embracing family and community within a Reform Jewish culture. I was given every opportunity to develop as a well-educated, caring human being. I loved playing with my golden Labrador, Shandy, starting my lifelong love of dogs. Shandy was my best friend, always there for me, comforting me when I was often stuck at home, missing school, parties or what seemed like all the fun events after having had one of my numerous stomach surgeries due to bowel blockages and adhesions; legacies from all the operations. Shandy always knew how I felt. He always understood, made me feel special and loved during those dark days of loneliness and pain.

When I was twelve, I decided to take up horse riding. My parents were dead against this, believing that it was a dangerous (and smelly) sport and that I had enough challenges to cope with, but nothing was going to stop me. I spent all weekend at the riding school in Totteridge, mucking out the stables and grooming the horses in order to earn an hour's lesson a week. I loved the heavy, musty aroma of horse and straw, the constant hum of teenage girls' chatter as we groomed, tacked up and lovingly tended the horses. There was a camaraderie, a shared passion for these magnificent animals. Some years later, I bought my favourite horse, Carnival, and he was stabled on a nearby farm along with two other horses, Caesar and Bonus.

One Saturday morning started like any other on the farm. It wasn't a show weekend, so we had decided to do a bit of training. I was asked to lunge Bonus, which involves the horse moving around you in a circle so one can observe their gait, help them burn off some energy and improve discipline. Everything was going well until suddenly Bonus threw his head up and, with mud and dust flying, pawed the ground with his front left hoof. Once, twice, three times he threw brown balls of earth into the air, eyes wild, nostrils flaring. I heard a heavy, loud, almost wild snort, and within a moment a thundering sound accompanied by four thundering legs came directly at me, knocking me flat in the mud. I was stunned physically and mentally. As I tried to get up, Bonus turned, snorted and pawed the ground once again, a crazed look in his eyes. Then he knocked my half-elevated body flat.

In that moment my parent's worries were realised. But there was no way I was going to let them know what had happened. I made an excuse and stayed with a friend for a few days in the hope that my wounds and stiffness would ease. It would be a year before I sought medical attention brought about by constant bouts of back pain and my limitations in being able to mount Carnival, let alone go for rides anymore or realise my dream as a professional rider.

Generally, I was happy growing up but for that significant part of my childhood when I was so unwell, struggling with stomach pain, back pain in my teenage years and a lowered immune system as a result. I regularly missed days, weeks and months at school. Over the years, those days of illness and missed social events and schooling translated into huge chunks of lost learning and a sense of being different – and not in a good way. I struggled at school, and remember many days and nights working hard on my homework, only to be deflated with a C or D grade. It was hard when I had missed so much of the basic tuition; it was like trying to build a house without firm foundations. I had low self-esteem – not a term that was invented then but I always felt 'less than', especially in contrast to Lorraine, who seemed to breeze through, rewarded with excellent grades for her efforts. I admired her so much, loved her beyond measure, and would have gone to the ends of the earth for her. To this day that unadulterated love is still present.

I know my family often felt frustrated with me as it seemed I was always spoiling some fun activity for them, Mum having to cancel things as I wasn't well enough to go because of stomach pains. I so desperately wanted to be well, but I don't think they saw it that way. I remember thinking they didn't believe me; they didn't think my pain, or my absolute lack of energy was real. I think they thought I was attention-seeking—oh if only they knew that was the last thing I wanted, attention for my sickness. I wanted to be well, to be playing sport and going to the parties and the outings just like everyone else.

I, nor anyone else for that matter, had any idea that my neural pathways were being set on a defective default setting, sending pain messages to my brain implying there was danger that needed to be protected by a pain message, when at times there was no new danger. That understanding had not yet become apparent in medical circles; it's only in the last decade or so that we have an appreciation of the impact of pain on neural pathways and brain messages. My early medical difficulties, regular surgeries and often excruciating pain experiences from my stomach and, later, my back injury had left my brain and body in conflicting states of dispute, no longer able to discern imminent danger from caution. I realise now that my back injury was further complicated by my limited core strength as a result of my many stomach surgeries.

I started to write and often wrote poetry – dark, sad pieces not to be shared with anyone, but my beautiful Shandy was always a good listener. My days of feeling alone and isolated were more than I felt was fair, but there was nothing I could do to prevent the felt stigma that my constant medical conditions caused me. I loved playing netball and table tennis at school and was good at both. I was in the school teams and those times were rare moments of feeling a sense of achievement, feeling normal and part of a team rather than the girl who was always ill. However, after 'the accident' my days of sport became progressively numbered as my back started to react to the impact of my untreated injury. I really missed playing netball and the whole team thing, so I decided to train as a netball coach. To my delight, I was encouraged by the sports teachers and I was the youngest person in the UK ever to qualify as a netball coach – a small compensation, but at least for a while it kept me in that wonderful team environment.

From late primary years through to my mid-twenties I enjoyed the company of a wonderful group of friends from my local youth group. We had so much fun together, enjoying weekly gatherings at 'the club' and weekends away. That time formed friendships that I treasure to this day. It was there that I felt a true sense of belonging. My parents were grateful for that, especially as they knew how tough school had been for me. Given the fact that I had missed about the equivalent of four years of schooling it was a wonder I graduated at all. But the school was so convinced of my limited academic abilities that they refused to support my application to university, an unprecedented move! I applied as an independent, a most unusual thing to do, and I was accepted into London University to study Psychology and Education.

I remember telling my parents that when I finished school, I would travel and study. My mother was all for the university approach; after all, I would have been the first one in our family to attend. My parents and I made a pact: I would complete my studies and then travel.

My first year at university was amazing. I made friends easily. No-one knew my history; I wasn't the one who was always ill. I was just like everyone else, excited to embrace a new chapter in my life and study subjects I enjoyed. But in second year, this changed. I was edgy and unwell. I couldn't sleep at night and became seriously agitated. I began waking up with more than just the usual aches and pains, anxiety and fireworks going off in my head. I developed a brain fog; it was like I'd hit a brick wall, but nothing could get me up and moving again. It transpired that I had a toxic thyroid which was playing havoc with my system. I was forced to take a year off university, spend three months sorting out the toxicity in my body and then having a thyroidectomy – yet another surgery and all that went with it. My university friends were now a year ahead of me so when I made the decision to go back my friendship circle changed. I didn't attend graduation and felt that it was all a bit of a nonevent. I received my graduation papers in the mail.

A pattern was becoming established, a slow and insidious pattern of pain that felt like every time I took two tentative steps forward, I ended up taking three steps back. I had always believed in 'mind over matter' but this pattern of periodic 'stops' in my life was making it a challenge to function normally.

# Reflections from this Chapter

- Living with underlying pain can compromise our overall health.
- Chronic pain almost always has a pattern – it's important to identify what that is for you.
- Not graduating with my peers was difficult. Our social networks are an essential part of maintaining a healthy mindset and when these are compromised, it's easy to fall into the depression trap.
- We often feel that just as we are 'getting there', another pain event brings us down. It's how we are supported to cope with that, and how we build our own internal resilience, which keeps us going.
- Pets are wonderful therapy to distract us from our pain.

# 3

# LIFE-CHANGING ADVENTURES

***The moments of happiness we enjoy take us by surprise. It is not that we seize them, but that they seize us.***
**Ashley Montagu**

In 1981, I graduated from university, and thankfully, was ready to quit my part time jobs in various sales roles. Pain had become my constant companion. Some days my mind was clear enough that I could hang out with friends and go on dates, but so often everything I did took effort and energy.

Despite this, after graduation, I left the UK with a friend to embark on a journey that was to change my life forever.

My stomach, for so long the physical reminder of my condition, now hosted a new family of butterflies as we planned our trip.

Although pain was my constant companion it was manageable for the most part of my new adventure.

We made our way through Australia, Malaysia, Thailand, India and Pakistan. Perth was our first stop in Australia for no other reason than we could only afford the ticket from London to Perth, not to Sydney or Melbourne. My part time work through university only allowed my finances to stretch so far! Within the first week we both found casual employment in sales which was to be our travel money later on. We also met a fun group of people on a boat trip and, during our four months in Perth, we shared many laughter-filled weekends together. We had a farewell dinner at Fast Eddie's in Fremantle and it was here that one of the boys from that initial boat crowd gave me a hug and a slightly lingering kiss on the steps of the restaurant. 'I'll come and visit you in England sometime,' he said.

Returning home after ten months of adventures, I attempted to settle back into life in North West London. I caught up with my friends, enjoyed a busy social life and bought my first home with a 100% mortgage. I also got myself a little black rescue dog, Mishka. She was possibly a mixture of Collie and Labrador, but I couldn't be too sure. I adored her and I took her with me wherever I could.

I was looking for work and my friend Jackie suggested I meet her employer. I hadn't really considered a career at this stage, just needed some work to get back on my feet. The interview went well, and I soon broke company sales records, selling matches and coasters for promotional use. It was a good start, but I struggled with the lack of mental stimulation in the job. In 1984 I joined another promotional sales company and became involved in both the sales and the buying from overseas markets. Mishka often accompanied me on appointments—she became quite the business mascot.

Even with all the stimulation of London life and enjoying the company and love of my family and friends, I felt like a square peg in a round hole. My friends couldn't relate to my travel experiences. My enthusiastic explanations of floating down the River

Kwai in a tyre for three days, camping on the riverbed, the smell of spices and incense muddled with sewerage and rotting food in India, descriptions of glorious Australian sunrises, and camping on deserted white beaches; all these wonders held their attention for no more than a polite five minutes.

My friends forgave my nomadic ramblings thinking I would soon forget and return to the more 'acceptable' life that revolved around work during the week and socialising on the weekends.

In contrast, life in London had a murky grey tinge. Margaret Thatcher was at constant war with the miners, there were strikes across the country, creating massive traffic and import challenges. Hooliganism was rife at the football stadiums and, on the streets, gang-warfare erupted between Indians and Pakistanis. The IRA was terrorising the country with indiscriminate bombings and the Global Economic Recession was starting to weigh heavily on the country. People were feeling the pain of a divided society, and fear was never far away.

Out of the blue, I started to have fits, sometimes full-blown and other times smaller moments of what I can only describe as 'absences'. It was like time stood still and nothing existed. And then I was back again, communicating as before, but with a heavy tiredness. I was frustrated, because here I was again, another 'health issue'; and doubly frustrated, because I couldn't predict when the fits would suddenly impose themselves on my life and ruin whatever I was doing at the time.

Here I was again, back on the medical merry-go-round. I tried to stay positive. Driving was becoming an issue because of the sudden onset of these events, no warning for me to pull off the road and wait for it to pass. I was diagnosed with a form of epilepsy that explained, or at least put a name to, the 'petit mal' and 'grand mal' fits. On reflection I probably had epilepsy years before, but it wasn't diagnosed until my early 20's.

My best friend Jackie had become engaged but during their engagement party Lewis felt seriously unwell and was diagnosed with Hodgkin's lymphoma. Not perturbed and forever positive, Jackie and Lewis married.

In September 1983, with my health once again transitioning into that phase of 'I'm feeling like life's back on track', I was looking forward to the Notting Hill Carnival, a spectacular street festival that begins in Notting Hill and parties through the Royal Borough of Chelsea and Kensington. This festival attracts over a million people every year and started in the mid-1960's in response to a problematic state of race relations in the UK. I and two of my closest girlfriends were about to leave my flat when we heard a noise on the staircase. There, climbing the last step toward my apartment, was a young man who looked oddly familiar.

'I told you I'd visit,' he said.

Standing on the last step to my apartment, smiling up at us was Dave, the guy with whom I had unexpectedly shared a kiss in Fast Eddies, Fremantle. He had arrived in the UK that day and was dropping in to say hi. As we had already planned to head out, we suggested he join us. I recall him telling me later that he thought all his dreams had been answered in one hit. Dave joined us that day at the Carnival and had a colourful welcome to London. I invited him to stay rather than head back to Earls Court to find accommodation.

It worked out well, so well in fact that, in May 1984, less than one year after he arrived in the UK, we married.

I was insanely happy, life seemed perfect. To make it even better, I had some wonderful news the day before my wedding.

I grew up with the knowledge that I couldn't have children due to all my stomach surgeries and health challenges. In fact, that had been the cause of a break-up some years earlier with a guy who I thought was 'the one'. He wanted a life with kids, and I couldn't blame him.

Dave, on the other hand, had a different approach. I don't remember his exact words, but they went something like; 'I'm not worried about the kids we can't have – I am happy with the woman I can be with'. That was such a beautiful gift and unexpectedly I was able to reciprocate.

The day before our wedding I received a letter with results from recent health tests stating that there was a possibility that I could give birth to my own biological children. You could not have found a happier, more complete bride-to-be on that day.

A year after we were married, we were discussing where we would like to raise a family. I was open to some new adventures, and so we decided that Australia was the place.

By this stage Jackie's husband, Lewis, was desperately unwell. His health had seriously declined, and Jackie was working fulltime which meant that Lewis was often home by himself. I thought about all the times when my health had robbed me of my freedom and how my beautiful dog Shandy had saved me. Dave and I were leaving England, so the decision was obvious. Lewis adored Mishka and, seeing them together, I knew just how much comfort her companionship would bring to his life, as it had mine.

# Reflections from this Chapter

- When dealing with pain it helps to look for silver linings, no matter how small.
- The love of a dog is a perfect antidote for bad days. Dogs rule – again!
- Pain can develop from a range of seemingly unrelated conditions, like anxiety, stress, compromised immune systems or maybe just change.
- We are more than our pain, and when we realise that it provides the opportunity to alleviate some of the discomfort.

# 4

# WHEN TWO WORLDS COLLIDE AND CREATE MAGIC

***And though she be but little, she is fierce.***
**William Shakespeare**

In 1985 Dave and I enjoyed an extended four-month journey back to Australia. We found work quickly, so it didn't take long to buy our own home. Of course, no home is complete without four-legged friends, so we adopted two black Belgian shepherds, Toby and Luanna.

I fell pregnant in 1986 and, for the most part, it was an uneventful, easy pregnancy, apart from one incident ten weeks before the baby was due. I was walking in the park with Toby and Luanna when they both came running behind me, knocked hard into the back of my knees and sent me skyward, knocking me flat on my back. Winded, I tried to get up and shake myself off. My back hurt, I was bruised and sore, but otherwise OK. But an hour later I started to experience severe cramps. Dave rushed me to hospital. The heavy landing in the park had sent me into premature labour. It seemed that my love for animals was always getting me into some sort of bother! It took two weeks of hospitalisation to stabilise me, but thankfully I continued my pregnancy and on 15 December, Dave and I welcomed our beautiful miracle daughter, Taryn, into our world. I struggled a bit (OK, a lot!) with back pain but figured that was to be expected.

My parents came over to visit six weeks after Taryn was born. After that, Dave and I agreed that somehow we would see my parents every year. To achieve this, we bought houses that needed renovating and sold them in order to pay for our next visit to the UK. It was the perfect market in which to do that and, combined with our well-paid jobs, we were managing life pretty easily for a young couple.

Dave worked in the mining industry and I had a few jobs, working in a childcare centre and selling promotional products such as caps, coasters, etc. However, it wasn't long before I felt the same lack of stimulation I had experienced in the UK.

One day I attended a business appointment at the WA Health Department. They were looking for caps and coasters for a health-promotion campaign. The minute I walked into that building, I knew I had to work there. The health environment felt right. I enquired if there were any jobs going for someone with my qualifications. Fortunately, a graduate job on the Quit Smoking team was being advertised in eight weeks. I spent those weeks swatting up on all the departments' projects and was the successful candidate. My life working within the health industry had begun.

On our next trip to the UK, we were proudly introducing Taryn to family and friends. A few days after arriving, I discovered I was pregnant again. Dave and I were delighted – how wonderful to share this news with my family face-to-face. Unfortunately, our news wasn't met with the enthusiasm we had hoped for. Mum and Dad were concerned, fearful for my health and not understanding why I would risk family in this way. My second pregnancy was the polar opposite to the first resulting in many complications. Despite this, during my pregnancy I enrolled in a Master of Public Health at Curtin University, Perth. It was a strategic decision, wanting to expand my networks in the field. I attended classes twice a week after work, taking Taryn in a stroller when Dave was travelling for his work. I went into early labour at 32 weeks.

Our second baby girl arrived, and we had four wondrous hours together. Then suddenly without warning, our tiny baby turned blue and flopped in my arms. Kara's heart was weak, and her lungs were underdeveloped. Oh my god – is this how my mum felt? Was history repeating itself? And worse still, I was warned, wasn't I! Guilt, so much guilt. What have I done? We were told that Kara's existence hinged on her ability to live through the next three years.

There were many terrifying times during that period: some in relation to Kara's constant hospitalisation and some to do with my physical ability to cope.

When Kara was seven months old, we experienced a particularly hot January in Perth, probably about 42 degrees. We had no air conditioning, so I was wearing a bikini because it was only the girls and me in the house. I never wore a bikini in front of anyone as I was conscious of my scars, my road map or 'flower' as the girls later called it. Dave was away on business and Kara had come home from hospital for a few days. She had feeding tubes attached to her as she was still too weak to feed normally. Taryn was sitting on the floor happily playing and Kara was getting sleepy, so I went to put her back in the cot. As I lowered her into the cot, my back completely locked, with my hand under Kara's little body. I was stuck in this position, bottom in the air, baby unceremoniously placed on the mattress. I managed to wriggle my hand free but that was about the only movement my body was going to permit. Copious beads of perspiration dripped onto my poor baby girl. I was terrified that she would drown in my sweat, or her tubes would block and cause her to asphyxiate. I had no idea how I was going to get out of this unseemly and painful predicament, but I had to stay calm somehow so as not to panic either of my babies.

Thank goodness for those days when the milkman delivered. Thankfully, all the windows were open because of the oppressive heat so I yelled and screamed for help.

'Hi there, could you possibly come and help me? I'm stuck!'

Poor guy. He found me, locked in bent double position over the cot with two screaming children needing attention. Undeterred, he carefully lifted me like a corpse and set me down on the sofa, still bent over, as I couldn't straighten my back. He called the ambulance. Everything went blank after that.

As was often the case in those years, my hospital visits were short, but the damage to my back was long-term and frustratingly non-specific. Over the next three years, I struggled with my often-unpredictable back pain, frequently exhausted from trying to manage the pain, be the best mum I could be to my daughters, work part-time and manage the household. Dave travelled for his work, which made it more challenging. Added to that, we worried about Kara and her fate, and even though she proved to be a little Aussie battler, we were in and out of hospital constantly over the three years, our funds quickly depleting due to medical bills. It sometimes took all my energy to stay positive on those occasions when I felt I was drowning.

Thankfully, Kara's health did improve, and our lives returned to that 'some-kind-of-normal'. Taryn was the more compliant one; Kara remained a challenge even on her good days. I have a theory that she had to fight so hard in utero and in her first three years of life, with so many painful medical procedures, often separated from her family that she developed a tough outer skin, often masking her real vulnerability.

# Reflections from this Chapter

- Life is a juggle – but it's amazing how we keep adapting and manage to get back on track. Living with chronic pain becomes a norm – so our brains become reinforced with the message that pain can become acute at any given, unwelcomed moment. It doesn't necessarily mean we are doing more damage to our bodies; it's just that our brain cells are developing new pathways which anticipate pain which in turn, creates the pain.
- Everyone has a different opinion—seek information, but ultimately trust yours.
- Staying positive is the key to navigating through the tricky times.
- There is always a funny side—it just might take a while to appreciate it. Humour is definitely one of the best therapies available.

# 5

# TWISTS AND TURNS

***New beginnings are often described as painful endings.***
**Lao Tzu**

In 1989, I started working part-time, working a five-day fortnight at the Health Department and continued my master's degree. Life was good, and true to our promise, we saw my parents every year, alternating between trips to the UK and them visiting us in Perth. My back was still giving me some grief, but nothing too alarming. A couple of years later Dave was offered the opportunity to relocate to Brisbane. We were delighted. The prospect of living in a more connected city, closer to the business hubs of Melbourne and Sydney, also opened more opportunity for me to progress my career. I started work with the Queensland Health department, and in one way or another that was my career trajectory for the following 25 years, working on a range of public-health programs and later focussing specifically on child safety.

Our careers took off. Dave travelled a lot for work and so did I. This meant that we sometimes 'child-tagged' at the airport, trying to balance our careers and family life as well as enjoying a full social life. I was passionate about my work and decided to expand my career, working as a consultant to the Mater Children's Hospital, during which time I also established my private clinical counselling clinic. My health was up and down and over the years I had more stomach and back surgeries, but these seemed to just fit around everything else. But at one stage, my back pain left me totally unable to move, resulting in more extended hospital stays and home convalescence. The specialist's advice was, 'I can't help you with your back as it's a complex situation and no surgery is going to help. You need to completely change your lifestyle, stop work and relax. But we can possibly do something to help your hip.'

I was devastated and infuriated at the same time. How could anyone reasonably expect me to stop work and relax? There was no way I could even contemplate this. I was in my late 30's, had young children, a blossoming career, a mortgage to pay and houses to renovate so we could go overseas regularly. I felt that the surgeon's suggestion reflected a total lack of understanding. The comment about my hip came as a shock. I hadn't even considered hip problems but the thought of something perhaps making a difference to my frequent pain was worthy of consideration.

It wasn't unusual for Taryn to ask if her friends could come over and talk to me about things that might be upsetting them. By this time, Dave and I had been foster parents for several years, offering emergency, short and long-term care to children needing some support.

In early 2001, when Taryn was 14, she arrived home with a classmate, Shae. We discussed some of the challenges Shae was facing in her life and agreed that she could stay overnight, after contacting her mum for permission. 'Overnight' metamorphosed into a challenging but wonderful three-year period in which we all learnt much about ourselves, our resilience, love and patience.

In that same year, Taryn decided to embrace Orthodox Judaism. She did this with a veracity of one totally and utterly committed. Then, at 20, the shock announcement that she was ready for marriage meant we had to involve the Rabbi in helping to find a suitable match. However, the timing didn't go quite how Taryn had planned. It had been about ten years since the conversation with the surgeon about my back and hip, and by now pain was controlling much of my life.

I could barely walk, let alone stand for too long; dancing at her wedding would have been totally out of the question. I wanted to be well and mobile for her wedding. So, my wise, understanding daughter gave me a wonderful gift. Time.

In 2006 I had a full hip replacement. Recovery was a long road, partly because hip replacements were not as advanced then as they are now, and partly because in my case there were further complications due to my complex back pain. Taryn was a fantastic help during those long months of recovery, and we spent many wonderful hours excitedly planning her special day.

On 27 June 2007, Taryn married Refoel, and I was able to dance at her wedding! If you have ever watched the movie or the seen the play, *Fiddler on the Roof,* you would have an idea of the wonderful party we enjoyed. Kara's school years were challenging for her and for us. Relationships were strained, but with love and perseverance, things started to improve. Kara graduated and embarked on a successful career. Shae, our foster daughter, rented a house with a few friends, worked in Brisbane and then travelled overseas while deciding on her career. Dave and I became empty nesters. There are of course many things that happen in life that can either make or break relationships. Moments when two people end up wanting different things. Goals change along with feelings and expectations. Sadly, in 2008, despite our best efforts, the dream of happily-ever-after ended for Dave and me.

## Reflections from this Chapter

- Lack of empathy from health professionals can cause long-term damage. Health workers may have the best intentions but may be quite siloed in their approach and not see the bigger picture of chronic pain management.
- Language is such a powerful tool. Many health professionals lack the training to recognise that their words, tone and body language can send either supportive or dismissive messages. We need our health professionals to guide us through the complex journey of living with chronic pain.
- With chronic pain, a holistic approach to care taking into account emotional factors as well as just physical is key to effective outcomes.
- The love of family is the most precious gift – if you don't have a

supportive family, then it's important to connect with friends or support groups.

- Try and find things to look forward to as this provides focus and strength.
- Emotional trauma, such as divorce, impacts our health physically and emotionally and can exacerbate pain. Take care to identify and deal with it. That doesn't mean your pain isn't real. It means that this stress activates the neural pathways in your already receptive brain and translates much of your emotion into a painful experience.

# 6

# ALTERED COURSES

***Sometimes the dreams that come true are the dreams you never even knew you had.***
**Alice Sebold**

Lost and all alone, I wandered through what was now my home, my four walls with empty, echoing spaces. I didn't expect to feel what I felt, the gut-wrenching emptiness, stomach strung so tight that I thought it would explode in my throat any moment. It's not that our separation was really a surprise; it had been heading in that direction for a long time. It's just different when it actually happens. And it wasn't just my marriage that had ended. The contract I had been working on had also come to an end, so I found myself without work, without a husband, and with children living interstate and overseas. Within a month, everything I had known and had been my day-to-day focus had disappeared. My husband, my income and any sense of me was lost. My future, how I was going to navigate this unknown territory, was completely unknown.

I walked into my home office, a stillness enveloping me. My body ached, from the inside out and the outside in. Pain was shooting through my back, my stomach had decided to join the tension party, and my brain was a fog of jumbled, half-finished, half-started conversations, regrets, fears and confusion. I sat down at the computer staring at the blank screen. I had no more excuses or reasons not to pursue something I had always believed to be the pinnacle of achievement, proof that I wasn't 'less than' everyone else. It was time to pursue my doctorate, to find a supervisor at the university who would be interested in my research question, one that had plagued me for many years working as a clinical counsellor and with child death data at the Mater Children's Hospital, Brisbane: the psychosocial impact of domestic pool drowning.

Two days later, I had a meeting at the University of Queensland and an agreement from the head of school to support my application.

The next forty-eight hours I hardly left the computer. I don't remember ever working that intensely, or excitedly. I was terrified that what I was writing would not be good enough. I had little to compare my work with and was unsure if my academic writing was up to the standard required for this level of submission.

I wrote, deleted, cut and pasted, researched and reformatted, and finally the document that had the potential to drive the next four years of my life was finished. I got up, paced the room, went downstairs, upstairs, in the garden, in the kitchen, ate potato chips and made copious cups of tea, all the while building up the courage to press the send key. This was my one chance, make or break.

SEND!

Little did I know when I sent my work into cyberspace that my research years were going to be my most challenging! I was totally blown away when not only did I receive a research grant through the university, I was also awarded a three-year scholarship from the Queensland Injury Prevention Council in acknowledgement of contributions to the field and the importance of this unique piece of research. It was happening, it was real. I felt I had a purpose again. But with all this excitement, my body was screaming. My back was giving me grief, slowing down my efforts to get on with life. I was frustrated: just when things come back into focus, when I feel a sense of joy, my body seems to sabotage every happy muscle, every glad cell. I had no idea at the time that emotions were so critically linked to pain, that stress is a precursor to pain, and that the overstimulation of my highly sensitised nervous system caused unnecessary pain messages to my brain.

Pain was never far away. There were times when I had to go to university to meet my supervisors and the journey was exhausting. Writing a PhD as a mature student is a stressful process, and there were times when I was dragging my body around in order to meet the requirements. I kept battling on, until one day, I realised the consistent, intense pain was contributing to me falling behind and having difficulty concentrating.

My supervisors were very understanding about the slower pace for my studies and accepted that this was my life, and we would get there in the end. I am very grateful for their support in that regard, and it was that attitude that made my PhD journey possible.

In the meantime, I had bought a little house on Russell Island, accessible only by ferry or barge. I rented out my house on the mainland and enjoyed most of my PhD studies overlooking beautiful Moreton Bay and enjoying the solitude that island living brings. It was an opportunity to try and slow my life down and probably, to hide a little from the world. I was tired. I was sad.

Two years later, friends invited me to attend a new course they had developed, Certificate IV in Facilitation. This was to be their launch and they were interested in my feedback, as I had spent many years of my career facilitating meetings, often contentious in nature. I was reluctant at first, still lacking in confidence and not keen to engage with new people. The unpredictability of pain flare-ups was embarrassing and my constant exhaustion managing the daily impost of chronic pain was tricky to manage. Having said that, a flicker of 'the old me' crept in, the me that loved new situations, new people and the opportunity to improve my skills. At the conclusion of the course, a celebration/graduation lunch was held in a lovely fish-and-chip shop down at Raby Bay, a classy canal estate in the Redlands. We were all feeling great. My friend mentioned that she had asked a friend, Neil, to join us for lunch as he lived on the canal estate.

Neil and I enjoyed easy conversation, and he mentioned that he still had a few days off work. Without a second thought, in my typical spontaneous way, I said, 'Well, that's a bonus. Why don't you come and visit on Russell Island? It's so relaxing, you can just chill out, read, go for a walk and I have a table-tennis table downstairs in the garage.'

The following day I met Neil at the ferry terminal. I could see him unwind almost immediately, shaking off the shackles of the city and whatever else was happening in his life. It was a comfortable, relaxed time for us and, when he left a few days later, we had both discovered an easy friendship.

We started to spend more time together, and I clearly remember staying at his apartment after many relaxed and happy evenings, having missed the ferry home. We enjoyed the uncomplicated situation – just friends, company with no strings attached. Neil would go off to work early, wave at me from the door of the spare room where I had slept, and politely wish me a lovely day. I always felt calm and happy in his presence, nothing was complicated, and life was good.

Over the next year, our relationship progressed to what I suppose could be called, 'the next stage'; a beautiful, intimate relationship. I was happy, my studies were at the interesting stage, and I felt I was being productive in that area of my life. I liked the balance and didn't spend any time looking further than where we were.

But, like all the best-laid plans, that too was about to change.

## Reflections from this Chapter

- Having a sense of purpose matters. Goals, however big or small, help us to know we are making progress.
- From adversity, great opportunities can appear.
- Sometimes, (almost always), slowing down is a good thing.
- There is often a strong connection with your physical environment and emotional state. Sometimes, changing your physical environment, even just swapping rooms in the house or repainting a wall can give you a sense of peace that can assist with emotional healing.
- A balanced life is a fulfilling life – and while that balance is forever changing, it's important to recognise the parts of your life that add

meaning and help you feel more complete.

# 7

# THE MORE THINGS CHANGE, THE MORE THEY STAY THE SAME

***Nothing changes if nothing changes.***
**Dawn Macintyre**

By 2011 my back was declining fast. Walking was becoming increasingly difficult and the unexpected attacks of pain were more frequent. I had trolled the medical merry-go-round, hoping to find some simple solution, but that wasn't to be. I was experiencing drop foot, a gait abnormality caused, in my case, from damage or irritation to the sciatic nerve. As a result, I found myself unpredictably falling to the ground in pain with little or no warning. I was exhausted and frustrated. I finally resorted to seeking advice from a neurologist and a surgeon and was scheduled for a lower-back disc replacement on my birthday. There was concern about complications because the plan was to go through my stomach, which by then had been subject to more than 15 surgeries, including removal of parts of my small and large bowel, a hysterectomy and bowel blockages. So, my stomach was nothing short of a complex mess of adhesions, not to mention the scar that looked like an international road map! I had also had a few more back surgeries by this time, including fusing and caging two discs in my neck.

Recovery from the disc replacement went well, and I really hoped that my back problems had been solved. Little did I realise that perhaps this was the trigger for far more trouble in the months and years to come. I don't know if that surgery had anything to do with my following years of chronic pain and acute flare-ups, or if my brain was receiving conflicting, inaccurate messages. Amongst the many diagnoses suggested was Failed Back Surgery Syndrome. I'm not sure if it even matters now; in fact, I don't think it does. I realise that my chronic pain is a combination of many elements; that searching for a diagnosis that fits all the symptoms is like searching for a white cat in a snowstorm. And it also compartmentalises the pain into one dimension when, in reality, pain is multidimensional.

In April 2011, Neil and I went away for a weekend to the Northern Rivers of New South Wales, two-and-a-half hours from home. We were blown away by the beauty of this part of the world and, driving around, we came across a stunning five-acre plot with magnificent views over the Eltham Valley. As we stood in awe, two white butterflies circled around me. My PhD involved working with families who had suffered the tragic loss of a child due to drowning. These families often spoke of white butterflies being a symbol of their child having 'passed over'.

That was it. We decided to buy the block of land there and then and create a combination of our home, a bed and breakfast, and free respite for families who were doing it tough due to life's circumstances. Highland Retreat was born that day. It had always been important for me to 'give back' to our community. I had, over the years, done a little toward this, and was honoured to receive the Redlands Community Service Award one year in recognition of my contributions. This was a gift, an opportunity, staring right at us. We purchased the land, had no idea how we were going to progress with the build, had the other property to sell, and of course, the minor issue of finding work in a new state. Spontaneity at its very best!

In March 2012, we returned to London and I was proud to introduce Neil to my family and friends. It was no surprise to me that he was a hit, his gentle, funny, warm nature captivating the love of my family and friends in an instant. They could see how happy I was, how relaxed we were in each other's company.

By now I was used to my back playing up, the pain being more severe at sometimes more than others. I hadn't fully acknowledged the incremental increase in pain and limitations to my activities such as walking, bending down or getting in and out of cars without wincing. It's similar to a child growing up; when you are with them all the time, you don't notice changes in them as clearly as does someone who hasn't seen them for a while. These things I had just learnt to accept as my 'normal', and I forget how the pain that slashes across my face tells all. Clearly, last year's surgery hadn't fixed the problem, and my friends' reactions to my diminished state and constant pain told all!

As always, when we visited the UK, we stayed with Lorraine and Les, my sister and brother-in-law. I vividly recall one incident when we were going into London on the Tube to see a musical in the West End. Although they would usually walk to the station, Les drove, as it was obvious the walk and a Tube ride to London was going to be too much for me. I always feel frustrated when things like that happen; it makes me feel so pathetic, frustrated at not being able to enjoy the simplest of walks. Excited to go and see *We Will Rock You* at the Dominion Theatre in Tottenham Court Road, we exited the station. Lorraine and Les walked on toward the theatre, chatting away, assuming we were right on their heels. I, on the other hand, was hardly able to put one foot in front of the other. Every step I took into the street sent shooting pains through my back. So debilitating was the pain that I cried out, grasping onto Neil to stop me collapsing onto the hard, unforgiving, wet pavement. I was lathered in perspiration, even though it was the middle of winter. I looked ahead as Lorraine turned in the distance, finally registering that we were not keeping up with them; but Neil sent them on, realising there was no way I was going to make it in time for the start, and not wanting them to miss out.

I did arrive, a gruelling half-hour later, exhausted from the effort of making my way just a short distance through the crowded streets to the theatre. I hated the stares I attracted; the offers of help kindly proffered by complete strangers made me feel even more self-conscious, a conspicuous, not-old lady shuffling along the street as if I was old and decrepit. I hated this! I can't say I enjoyed the show, because all I could think about was how I was going to get home again. Pain creates so much fear and, with it, alienation from the real world in a cocoon of terrifying anticipation; of making a scene, of screaming uncontrollably and at times, losing control of faculties so I end up embarrassed not only from the pain, but also from the unsanitary result!

I did make it back, but it was a long, slow, painful journey and one which changed my relationship with my UK family forever. It marked the beginning of years of constant rounds of debilitating pain flare-ups. No longer could I hide the fact that my pain was all-consuming and usually presented itself at the most inconvenient times.

Looking back now, I'd say that was the tipping point at which I lost confidence, and the start of when friends at home stopped making social plans with us. Too often I had to cancel; I couldn't be relied on to 'make it', to be pain-free enough to show up, let alone enjoy the party.

Over the next five years, my life withered into a pain merry-go-round, though it wasn't exactly merry! I was at a complete loss, feeling out of control, exhausted and frustrated. I couldn't trust myself anymore and I felt I had lost the essence of who I was. More dramatic incidents invaded and controlled my life, events that rendered me unable to move, unable to continue work, isolating me from friends and family, causing financial challenges, memory loss, opioid addiction, emotional and relationship confusion and a sense of loss and desolation that took me to such a depth of despair, I didn't want to live anymore. I had a private plan to escape this despair, and the plan was my comfort amidst the sea of pain.

I have thought about how to continue telling my story and I realise that what I don't want to do is spend the rest of this book sharing my journey in and out of hospitals, rehabilitation programs, doctors, specialists, etc. It was harrowing and boring for me, and I'm sure it will be boring for you. What I would love to do is share the insights I have gained from my experience of despair, intense pain, loss and confusion, to resilience and rediscovery. To creating my 'new normal'. This is MY story—we all have our own unique stories, different pathways to get to different places. My experience is just that, my pathway, but in sharing my story I realise there are many elements that us members of the pain tribe share that are often unrecognised or not validated.

But before we go there, I must complete the story of 2012. On our way back from the UK we stopped in Kuala Lumpur, Ipoh and the Cameron Highlands, a place of nostalgia for Neil, as he lived and worked in Ipoh in his younger years. Neil had organised a private candlelit dinner. It was to be one of the most memorable evenings of my life – in a good way. Waiters just for us, menus with our names inscribed, and a 'fire-lighting ceremony', all overlooking a garden alive with coloured lights and a clear night sky. I didn't think it could get much better. But I was wrong. In the privacy of this stunning setting, Neil proposed. At that moment, life was wonderful – I felt I would burst with happiness. Our relationship was so natural, so easy, and so exciting at the same time. I believed in us and our wonderful future.

Arriving back home in Brisbane, we enjoyed an evening meal at one of our favourite local restaurants. As we left, Neil staggered, said something in a mumbled fashion and dropped to the ground, suffering a massive heart attack. The following twenty-four hours were some of the most terrifying of my life.

When we arrived at the hospital, Neil was taken into a separate area whilst I completed some forms. About half an hour later, a doctor came out and suggested I call everyone I needed to, so they could say goodbye to Neil and offer me support in this difficult time. By what they could gather from Neil's condition, it had been too long since his first symptoms and they didn't expect him to last the night. I sat in shock for a moment, a cold chill gripping my throat. Neil's adult children live in New Zealand, and I didn't know them at that stage. It was Friday night, so Taryn's phone was off as she doesn't take calls on the Jewish Sabbath; and anyway, she was living in Sydney. Shae was overseas and Kara had just returned from the UK and was at a party catching up with friends she hadn't seen for almost a year. Thankfully, Kara had her phone within reach, and I was able to get hold of her. She came immediately, and then began the longest of nights, waiting in a lonely corridor, getting updates and trying to focus on the moment, my mind racing and frozen at the same time. Then a doctor arrived.

'We have the blood results back and things may not be as bad as we thought. Neil has had a massive heart attack, but we have organised for a surgeon to come in now. He is on the way, so we are prepping Neil for surgery,' he said.

Neil was in surgery for an hour while Kara and I sat in a waiting room near the theatre, almost pitch black, and no one else around. Silly, we didn't think to look for the light switch. We sat, comforting each other and holding hands.

Good news: Neil had stents put in to hold his arteries open. Bad news: he wasn't well enough for the triple bypass he needed so the plan was to go home, rest (as if he was able to do anything else, or I was going to allow him to!) and hope the stents stabilised him enough for surgery in four weeks' time.

Those following weeks were excruciatingly stressful. We felt we were living with a time bomb, ticking away, not knowing if or when it was going to explode. Fast-forward six months: Neil had his surgery, there were complications and the combination of the earlier heart attack and the surgical complications resulted in a lifestyle change for us both. From the outside it appeared that Neil had made a full recovery, but things changed that day forever. His ability to handle stress significantly diminished, a common occurrence apparently for people who have suffered severe heart attacks. Basically, his demeanour changed: there were lapses into depression and loss of self.

Enter Charli. During Neil's convalescence, our lovely Tibetan spaniel, Crosbie, passed away. Milly, his mate, had died the year before and suddenly the house was filled with emptiness and sadness. We lasted one night. We were on the lookout for another four-legged friend to bring that unconditional love and joy into the house, the cheekiness and distraction we so needed at that time. Within a week we found Charli, a tiny bundle of Spoodle fluff who sat in Neil's palm all the way home and stole our hearts from that day to this. We often say we should have called her 'Tonic', as she was without doubt the cure for those down-times. If you didn't know, a Spoodle is a cocker spaniel-poodle cross. Charli now has three brothers, Dougal the Cavoodle (Cavalier King Charles spaniel-poodle cross), Riley our Groodle (golden retriever-poodle cross) and Barnzy our Labradoodle. To be honest, I think she would prefer to be an only 'child' – she is a bit of a princess!

Life picked up after a while. Neil and I had moved in together just before his heart attack; I went back to my doctoral studies and clinical work, and Neil eventually returned to his work in finance. We had fun planning our wedding day, a marvellous distraction from our health challenges. On 4 November, Shae's birthday, Neil and I married amidst our friends; we even skyped our family in from the UK. The day marked a new beginning, an exciting future – although it turned out to be not quite what we had in mind.

Aside from our health challenging us both but also cementing our still-new relationship to a whole new level, we were about to introduce more challenges by moving to Northern New South Wales and commence building our dream home. There had been a dip in the real-estate market, and each time we tried to sell our Wellington Point house, the market seemed to drop a little further. So, we were chasing our tails and, when we finally sold, we ended up with a larger residual than expected. But in the scheme of things, with both of us working, we didn't see that as a problem. Neil had managed to procure a job as finance manager in nearby Lismore so, the day after our three-day honeymoon in Coolangatta, we drove across the border to the home we had rented whilst being close by to supervise our new build.

I continued with my PhD and, as I still had some clients in Brisbane, I went back three or four days a fortnight, staying with my daughter or friends whilst attending my clinic and meetings for my PhD at university. Driving that distance wasn't ideal; I was often struggling with the resulting pain from the journey, but at that stage, I had little choice.

During the house build, I had a particularly bad event with my back, and was confined to our rental home for six weeks. Across the road from us, in fact at the top of the road in which we now live, is an integrative doctor who has patients visiting him from all over the country. It took six weeks for me to be able to walk the three houses' distance down the road for my first appointment. As I shuffled across the road, I was lathered in perspiration from the effort. Two locals looked shocked at how different I looked, as the pain had written itself all over my body. I reflect now and can recall several times when I have seen 'that look' from people, friends and strangers alike. It sets up a different relationship, one of distance and fear, I think, as people don't know quite what to say or how to behave. In some ways, it's a bit like when someone dies; conversations can be stilted and awkward and, whilst people are usually sympathetic, it's not unusual for them to keep their distance because they don't know what to say. It's the same with chronic pain, especially nondisease-related, or non-specific chronic pain.

My experience with this doctor was weird. I stood in front of him fully clothed, and he stood maybe a metre away, assessing my posture and whatever else was important. He amazed me by referring to my stomach problems with as much, if not more interest than my back. I then lay on the table (that was no mean feat – it took about five minutes and multiple, muffled screams, for me to get onto it) and he lay his hands under my back and above my stomach, without touching the top of my body. He did this in a few different places, and then left the room. I lay there for a while then, after ten minutes, got up and asked what was supposed to happen next. That was it, he replied. I thought this very strange and couldn't see how this was going to be of any help. By the time I made it back home, I was exhausted and not at all sure it had been worth the effort. Fast-forward a few days, and I was more mobile; whether it was because of the treatment or because I was heading in that direction anyway, who knows? And again, does it matter?

I was frustrated that I was bringing pain into our new home, our new beginning. The following three years found me in an exciting new job, having to leave that job, in and out of hospital for 12 of those 36 months, and in total despair. I endured three more stomach surgeries, seriously debilitating back pain flare-ups which resulted in Neil having to care for me full time as I was incapable of being alone: I was unable to get to the bathroom without help, and even then, taking an hour to reach the en-suite just a few steps from the bed, all the while crying and screaming from the pain. Ambulance rides, long hospital stays, rehabilitation programs, pain clinics and pain programs, and what seemed to be endless search in the effort to find THE answer was the main feature of our lives.

I was a far cry from the woman who accepted that pain was her norm! This pain was beyond acceptable. The pain was exhausting. This pain changed me forever.

## Reflections from this Chapter

- Looking for a simple answer to a complex condition means you are asking the wrong question.
- Chronic pain is multidimensional – our body holds memories of past experiences which co-exist alongside current symptoms, making this condition a combination of past and present.
- Everyone's pain is unique.
- Chronic pain creeps up on you, before the sledgehammer hits.
- Chronic pain affects every aspect of your life. Broken sleep, exhaustion, anxiety and isolation are just a few

of the challenges that those of us living with chronic pain face on a daily basis. That can make us hard to live with – hard to live with ourselves at times and definitely hard for our loved ones.

- Chronic pain requires emotional resilience—and most of us need help in developing that. When you start to feel emotionally overwhelmed, consider reaching out to your doctor and discuss the best pathway for support. Maybe a professional counsellor or psychologist to help with the much needed emotional support, and perhaps getting into a pain management program will help with both improved understanding on how to manage your pain and offer the benefit of knowing you are not alone on this difficult journey.
- Everyone has a tipping point; however strong you are. You don't need to do this alone.
- Chronic pain can be a merry-go-round of emotions; despair, isolation, fear, guilt, financial challenges and having to

find yourself again. Be kind to yourself.

- I had to search for a 'new normal', a new Dawn if I was going to survive this. Find ways to search for your new normal.

# Part Two

# Escalation and Frustration

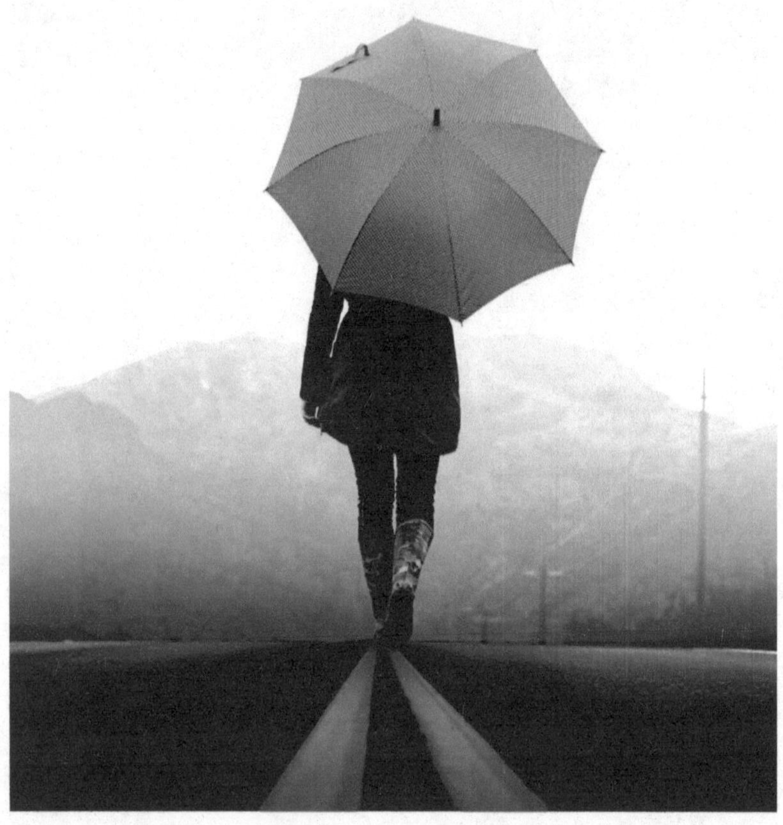

# 8

# WHEN THE PAIN TOOK CHARGE

***Most people don't want to die. They just want their pain to stop.***
**Lifeline**

In this section, I thought it would be useful to share some of the ways chronic pain has affected me. As I mentioned in *Part One,* everyone's pain experience is unique, but I have found some common themes which might help you and your loved ones understand and appreciate the challenges. It's important because so much about pain is hidden and that often makes the person dealing with chronic pain feel confused, fearful, lost and desperate. Because we don't live in isolation, the effect of our chronic pain has a flow-on effect to those around us. I thought the best way to illustrate some of the things I have lived with is to describe some of my experiences. Initially I thought to create separate sections, but there is so much overlap between the emotional, cognitive and physical affects that it seems less authentic to try and pull them apart in that way. What I hope you see is the enormous burden that chronic pain dumps on the sufferer and those around them: the confusion, the sense of loss, frustration and impact on the relationship with yourself and others.

I want to emphasise the fear: fear is a big one for me to conquer. Fear of the pain, fear of it limiting my life, of smashed hopes and dreams, of a belief that I am 'better'. Fear of ruining things for others, cancelling arrangements and causing them stress through my pain. Fear of changed relationships and fear of getting so tired, so worn down by the constant pain and the unpredictable flare-ups that I begin to doubt I am strong enough to go on.

Another frustration is a subject that really requires a book in its own right; the challenges of the medical system in dealing with chronic pain and offering timely and accessible pathways. In *Part Three* I'll talk a little more about that.

Remember, this is about my experience, and while it may be different for other people, my experience illustrates several common threads that chronic pain sufferers share. One key thread is the constant effort to try and stay positive while drowning in a murky sea of pain, brain fog and confusion. And of course, the desperate search for answers, to find that magic bullet that makes it all better. Now!

In early 2013 I found myself having to leave my new position as manager of a mental health program, as the pain was affecting my ability to move and my ability to think. My head was light, my brain felt scrambled as I grappled with trying to focus on my work whilst in constant agony and associated fatigue. I remember sitting on the wall outside of the office building, head in hands, tears rolling down my face, feeling broken. Just a few months before I had spoken to my insurance advisor and was on such a high, having started a new life, a new home and a new job. I was under a wonderful cloud of illusion – one of those intermittent times when I truly believed I could lead a 'normal' life of work and play. Neil and I had reviewed our finances and identified where we might reduce some expenses so we could try to reduce our new mortgage. Income protection – hmm, I was feeling great. Maybe I can finally ditch this? Boy, was I wrong! Thankfully, my insurance advisor gave me some very sound advice when I started the job. He looked at my medical history and was of course far more objective than me.

He suggested, rather than cancelling the policy, why not suspend it for six months and review it then? THANK YOU. His advice literally saved our home, although finances were still very tight. And as Neil is a New Zealand citizen, he was ineligible for carer's allowance. But that's a whole different story.

Within a year I had gone from a woman with energy, hope and vision, excited about the future, to exhausted, brain-fogged, frustrated and depressed, terrified of what lay ahead. The pain was ruling my life and Neil's. I reluctantly had to accept the fact that my lifestyle had changed. In fact, I was either bedbound or house-bound by this stage; getting into a car was impossible 90% of the time and, when I did, it would take a lot of manoeuvres, time and screams involuntarily exiting my mouth as I attempted to get into the seat. Then of course, I had to stay put for the length of the journey, a mammoth, exhausting, painful task. So, I was now at the stage of being unable to organise any social events, exhausted from sleepless nights of pain and days of frustration, limited movement and medication top-ups.

Where do I start? I mentioned before that I was someone who always looked on the bright side of life – sounds like a Monty Python sketch, I know! But it's true. Friends called me Pollyanna to the point that sometimes they didn't want to hear the positive side of everything – they wanted the validation of feeling terrible at that moment in time. I get it now.

Emotionally, I felt lost and alone. I was surrounded by love: love from my husband, my children and extended family. But I truly felt this was a battle that no one could possibly understand. I was grieving the loss of life as I had known it, the ability to manage the pain and continue to 'get on with my life'. My grief became an all-consuming emotion. I of all people knew that grief could do this to a person. My doctorate research focussed on the impact of grief and the gaps in support. I didn't realise at the time, but I was experiencing so many of the emotions that are identical to those who are grieving. Grief takes on various phases, and these include anger, frustration, denial, bargaining, depression and finally, hopefully, somewhere along the long, dark, seemingly endless, lonely tunnel, some form of acceptance. These 'stages' are actually a jumble of emotions, with no order to them and no luxury of warning. They just come, hit you when you least expect them, and bring you crashing down. You can fight them, you can accept them, you can fall in a heap while they tumble on top of you and consume you – but they are there. Learning to manage them is a process, one which takes acknowledgement, time, strength, energy and a will to crawl out of the despair. That's not easy when you suffer chronic pain because, most of the time, you are exhausted. And gaps in how health professionals can support us through the quagmire of pain became all too evident. In *Part Three* I will talk about how I believe support for non-disease-related, or non-specific chronic pain sufferers can be improved: what I needed, what I found and what I didn't find, even though I am a professional researcher. In the last year I have discovered there is a lot of information out there, but it's a disjointed mess with no well-documented, accessible central point. When you are heavily medicated, exhausted from lack of sleep and trying to get through another night and day of pain and your brain is a fuzz, it's no surprise that it's impossible to navigate the information.

This is a summary of my story from 2014 to 2017.

> By 2014, the pain was so debilitating, so dehumanising that I felt like I was losing my grip on life. And the pain monster found a new friend, a sadness monster, an isolated being who no longer looked, sounded or behaved like the

person my family and friends once knew and loved. It was hard to believe that I could become so medically pathetic and that the medical profession couldn't help me. It wasn't any wonder my family and friends doubted the truth of my situation. Well, maybe they didn't, but I had a fear that they did. After all, I had tried everything, and nothing was helping.

In 50 years, I had had more than 20 major stomach and spinal surgeries; between 44 and 59 years old, I had 25 hospital admissions. Each time I told myself that I would wake up a new person. That I would be free from not knowing when the pain was going to strike. You see, the old me, the 'then Dawn' was always positive, always believing that things will turn out for the best. But today, 12 June 2014, I hate that my bedroom is full of pain killers and bed pans rather than candles and pretty lingerie. The 'then Dawn' has disappeared. Yesterday was the day I decided I didn't want to live anymore. Somehow, I survived yesterday. Today I pray that I face a new beginning, yet I find myself facing more of the same. I can't shake that slow, insidious realisation that I have lost everything that matters to me – my ability to work in a job I once loved, my relationship as I had known it with my husband, the simple pleasures in life like enjoying time with family and friends, sipping hot mochas at sea-side cafes and taking long walks on the beach with my dogs.

I wanted my life back, but it had disappeared, teasing me with what was and mocking me cruelly with the remnants that were left. Now every day is a struggle. I sigh ... and drag my pain-ridden body upright and my legs over the side of the bed. My once-beautiful space now looms around me like prison walls. I am trapped here for long stretches of time, isolated, lonely and scared. Chronic pain has robbed my face of smiles once shared so easily. It has twisted my mind and body to the point where I barely

> recognise that woman staring back at me through the reflection of my bedroom window. Where did I go? Gripping the bedrail, I grit my teeth and dread the pain I know will come from standing. F.I.G.H.T. is here again. It doesn't matter ... It does matter. I don't want to live like this anymore, yet I am still here. FEAR – Fuck Everything and Run. But in which direction?

I had my 'out' planned by this stage. I had enough medication to 'do the deed', just go to sleep and that would be that. Simple, and being a scaredy cat, the least painful option! Looking back now, I find that so very sad. But I felt like such a burden to everyone. There was little joy in my life and my family were constantly worried about me. One devastating conversation was with my daughter, Taryn, who said she didn't want her children, my gorgeous precious grandchildren, visiting me because I was clearly in so much pain that she was worried how it would affect them. I was having so many flare-ups by this stage that it wasn't unusual for me to have an acute attack and end up struggling on the floor, vomiting from the pain and unable to hold back the screams and tears, as yet again I was helped back to the bedroom. On numerous occasions, I required an ambulance to get me to the hospital for significant pain relief. I get it, I wasn't a pretty sight and must have been scary for everyone. I wanted to be the grandma who could look after my grandchildren, give their mum a break and all those 'normal' things that grandmas do – but I was incapable. It had reached a whole new level and I was devastated.

Add to that the fact that I needed someone home with me all the time as the flare-ups were so constant. This limited Neil's life considerably. He never complained, but I felt this was so unfair on him. Our social life was zero. Thankfully we had created Highland Retreat, our beautiful home on five acres, so at least that was an outlet for Neil and a haven for our four dogs. In fact, it's probably fair to say that the few natural smiles I did manage over this time were when I was hugging the dogs or sitting outside with them, my bare feet on the soft grass and enjoying their unadulterated happiness running around the property. Barnzy, our labradoodle and the tallest of the four, had the most pats, purely because I didn't have to bend to reach him!

I was emotionally and physically spent, my spirit at an all time low. Medication and fatigue from the pain had robbed me of any intellectual pursuits. My search for answers took me to so many medical and allied health professionals and yet here I was, still stuck in the same rat trap and with no definitive explanation. It didn't help that expressions like 'it's all in your head' were stated – worse still, by a psychologist who supposedly specialised in pain management. And whilst now I know that means we can change our thought patterns, which in turn affect our pain signals, the context in which I heard these words did not offer that clarification. It wasn't until a few years after that experience that I was well enough to understand that messages to the brain can translate as pain even if there is no actual physical harm anymore. The pain signals are still flying up to the brain regardless. The pain is real. And in my case, as appears to be quite common with sufferers of non-disease-related chronic pain, there is neuropathic pain, which is enough to make the toughest of us scream. So, for us members of the pain tribe, the lack of specific diagnosis and the language used can leave us worried that other, non-pain sufferers believe:

- we are not really in pain
- we are making it up
- our pain is not real
- we are attention-seeking
- we can choose to change this.

And we are left feeling that:

- we are not validated
- we are not believed
- no one is prepared to help us
- no one understands.

It doesn't help that often the pain is invisible. From a judgement perspective, it's so much easier if you have a broken bone in a cast, or if you are in a wheelchair, because your physical state automatically signals you have something 'real' wrong with you. Chronic pain sufferers experience prejudice and lack of empathy similar to those in our population that suffer with compromised mental health, fibromyalgia, chronic fatigue and other autoimmune disorders. We can appear to be OK one minute and our world implodes the next. I guess for pain, those that really know us can tell by the strain on our faces, the artwork of fatigue and sadness that's etched like a painting of despair. Perhaps that becomes our altered state, the one that others no longer see as pain, but adapt to it being our 'new normal'?

## Friendships

Along with the pain comes fear. For me it was fear that I was going to make a scene and attract unwanted attention because of a flare-up. This happened often, both at home and while I was out. Let me share two of many such incidents. I referred to one of them as; 'Don't blame the pumpkin' to attempt to make light of yet another horrible situation.

I was excited but apprehensive. It had been more than 18 months since we had invited anyone over for a meal. I used to love entertaining; cooking something new and creative, chatting around our beautifully appointed kitchen as friends sipped their pre-dinner drinks and we caught up on our different worlds. Different, but over the years they had been the same. Our kids had grown up together, shared so many play dates, family times and excursions. We socialised together almost like blended families and our conversations knew no boundaries. But of course, all this changes as kids grow up and venture into the world. They create their own lives, families, friends and professions. So, it took a little more organising to get together friends, especially since our move to the Northern Rivers. The distance wasn't the problem when we first moved here. In our first year, we had lots of visitors and we also went to Brisbane often. I never allowed distance to be an excuse for not getting together with friends. But before that year was out, chronic pain and I created significant problems. I simply didn't have the energy to entertain anyone, not well-loved friends or family, and at times not even myself. I couldn't trust myself to be okay, to stand or hold a conversation, let alone prepare a meal remotely fit for consumption! The concoction of drugs I took each day played havoc with my mind, my body, my memory and my ability to put two coherent words together.

I was frustrated and bored with my life. I missed having a simple evening of friendship. I missed going out. Chronic pain had become the focus of my life. I hated it. Something had to change, so I bit the bullet and decided to invite friends over for a casual dinner. The thought of company made me feel a little happier. I began feeling a little more hopeful that life could return to me some modicum of normality. The burning sensation was still coursing through my back intermittently: the serrated knife feeling, twisting and turning, as it tried to navigate its way through the burning orange fiery tunnel it created. My skin still screamed with every touch and my head felt as heavy as a bowling ball perched atop a delicate flower. But this was a good day. I hadn't had a debilitating spasm for a few weeks. So, I guess this gave me the courage to want to enjoy some friendly company and lighthearted chatter.

I'd known Jo and Danny for years, and although they didn't truly understand the impact of debilitating chronic pain, they were thrilled to join us for dinner. They knew how rare an event it was for me to feel well enough to enjoy these simple pleasures, a sign perhaps that I was coping better than usual. The past two years had been filled with the misery and isolation that chronic pain brings. Realistically, I knew I wasn't up to anything too fancy despite being a decent cook. I knew the best that I could deliver was a casual evening of friendship. Nonetheless, I wanted a bit of the 'old Dawn' to shine through. I wanted to create a night to remember. I held this thought as I began setting the table with colourful Donna Sharam bush art coasters and placemats. Such a talented Australian artist, her work created an explosion of colourful joy across my table. I set a delicate spray of flowers in the centre of the table. I had bought them earlier that morning from the local Bangalow Farmers' Market. They created the perfect atmosphere – a warm, homely, welcoming space made for light-hearted fun and frivolity. My favourite bottle of Pinot Noir stood breathing on the benchtop. Two bottles of Pinot Grigio were chilling in the fridge and our elegant champagne glasses sparkled expectantly next to the plate of tasty looking pre-dinner nibbles. In my past life, my 'then self', I would have made these myself, but I knew doing so tonight would exhaust me, so I dropped by the local deli instead. Beetroot and hummus dips, crackers, crisps, cheeses, sun-dried tomatoes and olives created a colourful spread on the kitchen benchtop. I remembered to take the King Island Brie out a few hours earlier, so it was soft and not quite runny – just how I like it. I had been pacing myself, taking all day just to organise these little touches so I wouldn't wear myself out. I had my trusty list, an essential part of my daily activities these days, as my memory isn't exactly on the sharp side anymore! Pain is so exhausting, way beyond what I could ever have imagined. It's a cumulative thing, as the pain is always there, the tiredness just builds and builds, no relief. I had been living with this exhaustion for two years. I was exhausted from being exhausted. As the afternoon sun began to set, I gave in to the pain and took my usual afternoon rest. As my eyes slowly closed, I prayed that the rest would re-energise me.

By the time Jo and Danny arrived, I had put the pumpkin on the kitchen bench in preparation for one of my favourite accompaniments: a medley of roasted honeyed vegetables including garlic, sweet potato, potato and beetroot tossed in olive oil and harissa spice, with a drizzle of local macadamia honey to be added 30 minutes before the end of cooking time. We sat and had drinks. It felt so damn good to enjoy an easy friendship in our home and finally, a 'normal' evening. 'Chill' music was playing from our Spotify playlist. Candles were burning softly. The welcoming aroma of homemade simmered Thai tomato soup and bread fresh from the oven wrapped itself around the friendship. The fish was already prepared. It just needed to go into the oven. The night was perfect, I thought, as I looked around the room contentedly. Pictionary sat on the game table in the corner. I smiled at the image that came to mind of all of us playing together after our meal, doing things that normal people do.

With my first glass of perfectly chilled white wine swallowed, it was time to cut the pumpkin. The smile that beamed across my face disappeared the moment I found my feet. That all-too-familiar pain filled my face. Momentarily, I braced and screwed my fist into a tight ball. I steadied myself as beads of sweat formed on my brow. I held my breath, willing the pain to subside. I could feel Jo and Danny staring at me with concern. I smiled determinedly to avoid any conversation about my pain. Nothing would ruin my perfect evening. I put on my well-worn mask of serenity and sparked up some light-hearted banter. The pumpkin was waiting on the chopping board. Surprisingly, I made it all the way to the kitchen bench. I was so pleased with myself as I raised the knife to cut the green slightly stripey skin of the pumpkin. I'd barely moved an inch when it happened.

My world was instantly filled with a burning electric sensation, consuming my whole being, sending bright red, burning, warning signs through every nerve and fibre of my body. I manically grabbed the benchtop. From nowhere I heard a guttural scream that sounded like a wild animal caught in a trap. It was me. My head spun, my knees buckled, and my jaw clenched as I hung on to the bench for dear life. I heard chairs scraping from across the other side of the bench, a swampy haze of noise confusing the scene. What a sight I must look. Fuck, I can't believe this is happening – not again, please, please, not again!

Another searing bolt of electric current and I let go, ending up on the floor. I was in such despair until I felt the solid comforting arms of Neil gripping me under my armpits to try and get me to my feet. Tears streamed down my face. Pain struck me like a bullet exploding through my back and along that familiar pathway of nerves throughout my body. Neil did his best to help me into the bedroom, having no choice but to half-drag, half-carry me. Screams mingled with gasps as I fought to breathe through the pain. I tried to stand. I tried to walk and make a more graceful exit. I tried to keep some sort of dignity, but I was helpless. My movements were excruciatingly slow – my exit far from graceful. Ten minutes felt like ten hours.

What was I thinking? There is no grace in pain. Sweat streamed from every pore of my body. I fell several times to the floor, a pathetic ragdoll. I grabbed at anything to get leverage, but the kitchen cabinets were all too shiny and this made them slippery. The pain brought a lump of bile to the back of my throat. I felt myself convulse and dry retch. A warm wet puddle dribbled from my withering body onto the kitchen floor. It couldn't get much worse, but I knew it would. Who was I kidding to think tonight would be any different? I pitied myself but felt guilty at the thought. Pity and pain mixed like a toxic cocktail in my mind. Neil, to his credit, finally managed to drag my wretched body into the bedroom. Carefully and as gently as he knew how, he guided me onto the bed. Between my agonising screams and tears, I bit my lip, trying to minimise the horror scene I had already created, desperate to find a comfortable position. The darkness of pain reached out to me, enveloping me in its embrace. I desperately needed to use the toilet (again), but it was all too much. That's a cruel twist – the pain stimulates the nerves, which stimulate the feeling of needing to go to the toilet. But that's far too much of an effort – impossible to get there. I was physically and emotionally spent. I had nothing left for the journey that would take five agonising paces to get from the bed to the ensuite. I couldn't move. In despair, I felt my life was so unfair. I vaguely heard the hush of voices outside my room and my name carry across the room amongst the otherwise indiscernible chatter. Jo and Danny were clearly distressed with what they had just witnessed. I wished I could reassure them, but Neil would have to be the life of the party now, such as it was. After all, it didn't make any sense to waste all that good food. There was no point in everyone else going to bed hungry.

The pain was incredible. I prayed it would pass but I knew I was being unrealistic. Every breath sent a fresh explosion of burning bullets throughout my body. I envisioned myself as a circuit board of millions of wires, all electrified, all short-circuiting as random acts through my body. I saw this in colour; in gold and red, like rivers of molten gold and dark crimson blood chasing each other through the millions of pathways that make up this wretched vessel of mine. Neil kept popping his head in to see if I was ok. I'm not sure what he expected me to say. I couldn't talk, anyway. The pain was too consuming. I pathetically waved him away to re-join our guests. It was embarrassing enough without both

> of us leaving the room. I began feeling waves of depression wash over me. I had tried so hard to have one 'normal' evening: to do what people do, make a meal, enjoy the company of friends in our beautiful home. I was wracked with guilt for ruining yet another evening.

Unfortunately, this was not an isolated incident. There were many similar occasions (although I went off pumpkin for a while!) between 2013 and 2016, when I thought I was Ok to make plans. Invariably they ended either with me in hospital, in intense pain, or having to cancel. Shopping centres were another challenge. This next scenario describes another occasion when I was determined to be OK and it didn't pan out. This was in 2016.

> I managed to convince my friend Donna to take me to our local shopping centre so I could get out and about, do something normal, sit and have lunch together after she finished her shopping. I hadn't been able to drive for a few years by this stage, so even if I

did feel up to getting into a car, I had to rely on someone else to take me. I was also constantly fearful of having a flare-up in public and didn't have the confidence to go anywhere alone. I know I was catastrophising in my head, ('catastrophising' being another of those words, so often used professionally, that leaves us pain sufferers feeling judged), but my experience didn't give me any other guidance as to how to prepare for each moment in the day. I gingerly positioned myself in the car, firm cushion behind my back so I could stay as upright as possible. Donna was looking concerned. At that point I said to her, 'Please don't keep asking if I'm OK. I'll tell you if I'm not.' I hoped that would ease her mind, and we chatted on the way to the shops, a 20-minute ride that admittedly caused me significant physical discomfort. But it was oh so good to be out and about.

As I followed Donna into Woolworths, we walked slowly down one aisle. I began to tense. I felt

I was in trouble but didn't want to ruin our outing. Just regular shopping for Donna, but for me, it was a big deal to be out with a friend and back 'in the world'. Deep aches and burning sensations were flying through my body and I started sweating as we walked along the frozen-foods aisle. I lifted my chin, looked straight ahead and put my next, obviously not my best, foot forward. As I did so, right in front of the frozen peas, I staggered as the pain attacked my back and legs and caused me to grab onto the trolley. I couldn't right myself, couldn't straighten and the trolley started to swerve. Donna thankfully grabbed it as I tried desperately to pull myself together and be upright. But my body had other plans.

I fell to the floor, but that position was agony, so I tried to get up again. By this time, a crowd had gathered, and a kindly member of staff offered her assistance and to call an ambulance. I adamantly rejected the need for an ambulance, knowing what a spectacle that would create as well as the now-well-experienced fact that, once in ED, the same merry-go-round of questions, medication, waiting, etc. would occur. And of course, the worry for Neil. So, I asked for a chair and there I sat, in the middle of the frozen-foods aisle, people shopping around me until I could relieve the pain with some medication I had with me and, I hope graciously, accepted the help of three staff members back to the car. The staff were great, Donna was concerned, and I felt like the biggest party pooper ever. Yet again, I felt that familiar guilt, the betrayal of my mind and body in believing I could be 'normal'. In my mind, I had ruined what should have been, an enjoyable time with a friend. And Donna came home without her shopping!

What followed from that incident was my belief that Donna was reluctant to go out with me again (understandably) and another kick to my confidence that I could cope with going out. I didn't trust myself anymore. I know I should have paced myself better, maybe just waited at the Coffee Club while Donna did the shopping. It's so hard to slow down when you are hopeful that things will be OK. I tried to reconcile these events; attempted to be realistic and accept I had to pace myself, but it left me fighting depression, a sense of uselessness. I struggled to see how my life was going to improve. And I felt my friend had lost confidence in being with me, as well as any joy. I was a burden – again. I later found that Donna didn't feel that way, but I know that it has taken a few years for her to be confident enough for us to go out and 'have fun', to trust in me to pace myself.

## My Family

Apart from the theatre incident I mentioned in the previous section, there are a few other stand-out events. As my parents, siblings and extended family live in the UK, I try hard to shield them from the reality of my pain and to focus on the good things happening in our lives. They didn't need to know about all the challenges we faced; my parents are amazing and the last thing I wanted to do is give them cause for concern. As a parent, I know just how helpless it makes you feel, unable to protect your child and take the pain away. And my siblings; well, they probably had enough of my health interfering with their lives when we were kids, so I didn't want to be that person anymore. Sometimes, though, we don't get what we want!

We were in the UK, having enjoyed a house-sit for a few weeks just 30 minutes from my sister's house in Pinner. I always miss my dogs when I am overseas, and housesitting is a great opportunity to have some canine company and give Lorraine and Les a break from us invading their home for extended periods. On this occasion, we were due to leave the house-sit and return to Pinner. My back had been tetchy for a while, but I was managing. Neil had carried our things down the stairs, and I was just giving the upstairs bathroom a wipe over when IT happened. Cascades of fire ran through my back and sweat seeped from every pore of my body. As the familiar motion of collapsing legs drove my body toward the floor, I grasped the sink as my mouth released an agonised wail. Spasms invaded my muscles and my nerves were having a riot, trying to compete in the extreme-agony stakes. As I tried to breathe, tried to move, muscles and nerves conspired to defy my brain and win the battle of pain and immobilisation. In short, I was stuck.

Neil came running upstairs but was unable to move me. We were in a real pickle, having to leave the house, yet not knowing how that was physically possible. I absolutely didn't want an ambulance, so Neil called Les, who is a tall, fit man, to seek his help. I barely made it through the next 45 minutes waiting for Les to arrive, terrified as to how I was going to get out of this mess, so scared of the pain, yet trying desperately to calm myself.

The next two hours can only be described as a macabre circus act. No one in my family had seen me in quite this state, and I think Les was expecting something far less severe than what confronted him. He was in for a shock. Coming up the stairs with Neil, both men assumed they would be able to support me down the stairs. But that wasn't even a remote possibility. As they touched me, my body screamed in fury and, again, guttural, bestial sounds escaped from my deepest being. The frustration, embarrassment, pain, sense of helplessness and uselessness overwhelmed me. I felt like a tortured animal trapped in a cage, yet there was love around me. I was so confused. So helpless.

Apparently, it took an hour to get me down the stairs; then the challenge was to get me into the car. We laugh about this now, but at the time it was horrific. Two grown men, holding a 176cm screaming woman parallel to the ground. Car doors open – they attempted to slide me across the back seat as I screamed in pain. The weird thing about all that is this was a town-house complex with a few hundred homes within a small area. Not one person, not one, came out to see if I was OK, or was being abducted. Don't you find that unsettling?

Anyway, we got back to Pinner and, somehow, they got me to bed. At times like this, I was always desperate to go to the loo because the nerve endings become stimulated – but too often, this bodily function fails to wait instruction; hence, a major embarrassment. I guess Neil had got used to that, and at home we had all the things needed to deal with these events. But not here, not in my sister's house in Pinner. Please no!

A few interesting things came out of that event. Les admitted to never having realised the extent of my pain and said he 'found his empathy gene' after the experience. In a way, that was validating for me – not that I wanted to announce my situation to all and sundry, but it did help them just a tiny bit to understand the challenges Neil and I go through when we cope with this back home in Australia. I always understate my health situation when we speak on the phone, usually saying I'm fine unless I'm in hospital, and obviously not. I guess this gave me a sense of 'okayness', of validation that they didn't think I was exaggerating. When I did say I wasn't doing too well, I think they now realised it meant I was pretty damn off the scale in pain.

One other outcome from this event created mixed feelings. My parents came over and sat with me for many days, my mum, bless her, desperate to feed me chicken soup, the well renowned Jewish panacea. Not only was I vegetarian, I was unable to sit in a position for over a week to even drink soup if I had wanted to! I hated to see the pain on their faces as they witnessed my pain. As a mum, I can really feel how that must have been. And they had been through all of that for so many years when I was a child, I felt so guilty bringing it all back to them. On the plus side, Mum and Dad felt relieved that they could be with me during this time because of course, when we are in Australia, they feel helpless.

There are many family incidents I can recall, but the sum of all of those is that, in my eyes, I became a burden to my children and an unfair concern to my parents. I was unable to support them as a mother, to help with the kids or even just visit for a coffee, lunch or whatever. The tables had turned, and I was the one they felt they had to look after. I lost all sense of pride, my position as the adult, the protector. Here they were, here everyone was protecting me when that was most definitely, the last thing I wanted.

## Neil and I

I was feeling very sad, lost, and my sense of self had taken a massive hit. Guilt played an enormous part in this emotional roller coaster, particularly in relation to Neil. Our relationship changed. Our newly married life, full of excitement and adventure, now felt like a distant dream that I had to consciously call up to remind myself how it could be again. But that attempt at visualisation caused emotional trauma, because I no longer believed we could be that couple. I felt I had cheated Neil, given him a bum steer, and now he was stuck with some useless woman who was practically incapable of laughing or putting together a whole sentence. The medication I was on was very strong, yet it wasn't helping. What it was doing was causing memory loss, slurred speech and an inability to hold a sensible conversation. And yet a year or so before, I had gained my PhD. This was so unfair!

One thing that was never spoken about in all my appointments with the GP and in the pain programs I attended was how this constant chronic pain affects our relationships. Apart from the financial stress created because I couldn't work and Neil had to be home to look after me, our conversations and our physical relationship changed.

I didn't want to keep saying I was in pain, but I didn't have to. It was etched all over my face during the day and, more times than not, seriously restricting my movement, keeping both of us awake at night as I struggled to find a comfortable position. I could see his concern, and of course, he frequently asked if I was OK. Inevitably, I wasn't OK, and I started to get frustrated with him asking. I wanted him to go out and do some things for himself, but he was afraid to leave me, and to be honest, I was afraid to be alone. Seeing the concern on his face was awful for me, and even worse when I was hospitalised and in rehabilitation. His life was centred around me the whole time, and not in a fun way.

When I did feel capable of doing things, like making a cup of tea or hanging out the washing, which was a good stretch for me as long so Neil carried out the basket, he would jump into action and want to do it for me, concerned that the movements would trigger another ugly scene. And at times they did. It took me two years to be able to pour water from a kettle or take a one-litre milk carton out of the fridge. The action of lifting and tipping caused a ripple effect and spasms through my body. Nowadays I tilt the kettle with the base still touching the benchtop – a simple adaptation I learnt whilst trying to develop a modicum of independence and to minimise the risk of spasms and flare-ups. We were caught between loving concern and enabling behaviour which further limited my confidence and activity.

Physical touch was as big a challenge as the emotional situation. Neil was scared to touch me in case he hurt me, and I was scared for him to touch me. Most of the time my skin was so sensitive, touch was like a burning sensation. For a hug, well, it's not exactly pleasant for the hugger or huggee if the person being hugged grimaces and tries to grin and bear it. But I expected him to read my mind. On occasions when I felt I wanted physical touch, he of course couldn't know unless I told him. But I unreasonably I expected him to just know, so even when I felt that way inclined, it was stilted at best.

As to anything more intimate, forget it! Perfect for a newly married couple – not. There was no way I felt like having sex or had enough energy to even contemplate it. Even if I wasn't totally exhausted most of the time, how was I going to find a position that wouldn't be painful or, worse, cause me to end up back in hospital? It was a vicious circle of fear and pain, and we had to try and navigate that quagmire every day.

And to make matters worse, the pain, the medications and my history of stomach surgeries resulted in blockages, constipation and incontinence. I have very little core strength as a result of these surgeries, so that doesn't help with strengthening muscles. The pressure when trying to go to the loo often caused intense back pain; ultimately, I had to have surgery to fix my prolapsed bowel. I was feeling unattractive, useless and sad.

Communication was a major challenge – and yet here I am, a trained clinical counsellor who has spent my professional life supporting others in navigating difficult situations using effective communication methods. Like many couples, Neil and I deal with things differently. Neil closes down and is very private. I, on the other hand, want to talk about things, to share them and try to understand. I know Neil just wanted to 'fix it' for me and was very frustrated that he couldn't do so. We had to learn a new way of communicating our needs – and over time, I am proud to say we have done that well.

In *Part Three* I will give some examples of how we navigated this tricky communication process.

## Some hospital experiences

Hospital visits were frequent over this three-year period. We are incredibly fortunate that, even though we live in rural Australia, we have a fantastic ambulance service, and I admit to having put them to the test on many occasions. Poor Neil. He always had to make the calls amidst my protestations, yet reluctant admission of no alternative. I was incapable of speaking through the pain, so this task fell to him; I blamed him, yet he was my rock, my protector. Over time we, or rather, Neil, had everything organised like a well-oiled machine. Whatever I needed for hospital was in easy reach and I had my 'hospital bag' always at the ready. The following is one example of the many difficult home-to-hospital transfers.

> I had taken the big step of meeting friends in picturesque Lennox Head for lunch. I had been feeling quite good for a while and was confident this was going to be a great afternoon. These friends had been living overseas for many years and it was lovely to be sharing time together locally, knowing we had years ahead of us to enjoy similar experiences. They were unfamiliar with the area, having returned from their extended overseas sojourn to live in Brisbane.
>
> Excited to walk with them on the beach and share some of our local culinary delights with views to die for, we met at the beach, parked our cars and started a gentle walk on the glorious golden sands, the sun gently warming us, the wind brushing our face, and the sand warm between our feet. It was

so good to be sharing this together. I was a little slow with my walking, feeling tension in my back. Whilst my slow gait had become normal to me, my friends were displaying signs of concern as they slowed their pace to stay with me. That 'look' that I had come to know well, always accompanied by THE question – am I OK? Chatting away and trying to push their concerns aside, we continued to the café strip. As I took my next step, my worst (now familiar) nightmare decided to launch itself squarely on the high street, in front of 'the world'.

My back spasmed, I couldn't stand, and I let out an involuntary scream. Sweat started seeping out of every pore of my body as I tried to maintain an upright position. Not so lucky. Grasping my friend's arm, I slithered south, only to find myself in the hellish 'caught between' motion of unable to stand, and unable to go down. I vomited, lost control of my bladder and wanted to disappear. People gathered round, some saying they had called an ambulance, others telling me to have faith in Jesus (yup, you heard that right). And at the centre of that commotion was a most unwilling, embarrassed me!

Neil came to my side. I wanted to die of humiliation. I wanted to get off this rollercoaster of pain. 'You didn't sign up for this,' my eyes appealed to him. He took my hand and quietly reminded me, 'We're in this together'. Grimacing and overwhelmed with frustration, I tried to slow my breathing. Just breathe, Dawn. Neil knew it was pointless to suggest going to hospital, always the very last option on my list. I thought if I could just have a strong pain killer then perhaps, just perhaps, I could get home. I popped the medication I always carried with me into my mouth, grateful for the water the manager of the IGA had bought to me. I just wanted to get home, to disappear. Yet another ruined attempt at 'being normal', at going out with friends.

I insisted I didn't want an ambulance, so desperate was I to avoid yet another hospital event. So, beautiful, kind, considerate people stepped into the middle of the road, stopped the traffic, and somehow Neil and our friend managed to lift me into the car as screams involuntarily escaped my lips and a shroud of pain and embarrassment devoured my being.

Somehow, we got home, a painful 30-minute car ride no longer unfamiliar to me. I was determined to get to my bed, to have this over with, take whatever I needed and wake up better in the morning. But I had already taken my strongest prescription meds and they'd had no effect at all. I wanted to force myself somehow to believe there was hope that I could get through just one night and it wouldn't end up the same as other nights. But it wasn't looking good. Still insistent that hospital was not going to happen, Neil suggested he ring the doctor when it became obvious I was not getting any better. I had to concede, hoping they could come out, give me a magic something and the world would improve. But that was not how the plan unfolded. He was told our house was located outside their catchment area for home visits.

Left with no choice, and despite my now weak protests, Neil called the ambulance. He went into the well-worn routine to put the dogs away in their garden so that there was clear access for the ambulance that would soon arrive. He dragged out my blue cabin bag, ready to pack with my 'hospital gear'. Nighties in one place, toiletries in another, my spare phone charger, my Kindle and thyroxine medication – and Neil at the ready to open the door for the paramedics.

Sometime later, they arrived and, again, despite my feeble implorations to just fix me where I was, they began to prepare me for the journey to the nearest hospital. I wanted to convince them I would be okay. I wanted to be like normal people who kicked their toe and cried but got up and going again. I wanted to plead to stay home but I knew I was beyond pleading, no energy to fight. I was far beyond being able to manage anything on my own. I knew I was going to hate this. I was hopelessly fighting but not winning. The word 'Fight' became an acronym for what was to happen next - Fuck, I'm Going to Hate This!

Talking was too much of an effort through the pain. I broke into hot and cold sweats, terrified about the moment the paramedics would move me. I knew that would spark yet another explosion of bullets coursing through my body. I was trapped between agony and despair. The paramedics had called for back-up, having assessed the severity of my pain and potential challenge of moving me. I had fallen into a wild and hysterical panic that made it hard to breathe and calm myself. No straight morphine for me: I'm allergic to the usual 'go to' medication for severe pain. The paramedics administered some other Valiumbased drug then waited. Ten minutes later, two more paramedics arrived. Together they attempted to lift the gurney with me on it. I was sleepy, but the moment the gurney moved I screamed in agony. The drugs had no effect, so they suggested administering a hallucinogenic drug called ketamine. They explained it would give me an out-of-body experience but allow them to move me without pain. They told me not to worry and that I would be safe. It was overwhelming. Even in a drug-induced state, I was fed up and desperately sad. I hated my life. I felt like such an imposition on everyone, even the paramedics, but I was grateful for their attention. I just hated the thought of needing it. This all marked me as the lost Dawn, the pain Dawn – oh where oh where had the 'then Dawn' gone?

Feeling like a helpless child, I allowed them to administer the ketamine. It took seconds to kick in and when it did, I felt the room tilt as the lights around me danced. It was just like a scene in a Hollywood movie. I heard faint, distorted voices bouncing off the walls around me; strange faces staring through me, elongated, green and wide-mouthed. Voices became distorted. Ghostly figures moved around my bed seemingly in slow motion. Neil's face was inches away, but it had become a long, rubbery mask. His contorted mouth told me I was going to die as he held my shoulders down. His words filled me with terror. I screamed again. In the next moment, I felt their hands upon me. The ghostly figures were taking me by force, with no care for my pain and suffering. Suddenly the air changed. I felt a cool bristle brush across my skin, and bright lights blinded me as I felt myself floating toward an illuminated box. It was the ambulance, but at that point it looked more like a spaceship. Inside, the ghostly figures connected me to tubes. I tried to protest but my mouth refused to form any words. I didn't see Neil. Perhaps they took him.

Had hours passed? Days? I had no idea.

Voices floated in and out, slowly beginning to make sense as they whispered words of reassurance. The ghostly figures had gone, along with their illuminated box, as the inside of the ambulance slowly came into focus.

Where am I? I tried to speak but the words stuck in my throat. Had I been dreaming? I wasn't sure. Then vaguely I started to remember someone saying something about a ketamine injection. The sheet felt wet beneath me as my connection to reality returned. The ambulance tilted, and with it, the familiar explosion of bullets of pain. Help me! I shouted but not a sound was heard. Why couldn't they hear me? Where was Neil? I felt so disorientated. I wasn't sure how long those moments of relief had lasted but the pain monster had well and truly returned with a vengeance. I tried to move my hands, to signal to the paramedics that the pain was killing me.

'Calm down, breathe, relax', I heard them say as they began moving the gurney out of the ambulance and into the hospital's Emergency Department.

Reality kicked in and, with it, the horrendous thought of returning to hospital, my third Emergency Department visit in 18 months.

Fourteen hours later I lay in the same state, with every breath bringing a fresh wave of pain. Emergency staff rushed past, stopped momentarily to look at my chart, then left. Clearly someone else was more important, and I understood that they are bound by priorities; but to me, my pain was priority. It was excruciating. I started to feel betrayed, that I was 'less than' everyone else. My pain was real, but no one seemed to hear that. I desperately wanted them to listen. Their faces told me they didn't believe me. If only I could tell them I wasn't faking it.

If only I could show them my pain was real and consuming. Where was Neil? I had no idea. And then suddenly, he appeared. My champion, my saviour.

'They don't hear me, Neil,' I cried in frustration.

'They don't believe me.'

'Ssshhh it's alright, it's OK,' he comforted.

Neil stood by my side, unable to convince anyone who cared to listen that I was not some ranting lunatic. His presence was comforting nonetheless and reassured me that at least someone could hear me.

'Thank you,' I whispered to him.

This awful situation went on for two days, with me sidelined into a small area off the main emergency ward. I was frequently topped up with drugs that did nothing to ease my pain. Neil was so frustrated seeing me like this. He felt as helpless as I felt traumatised. I did everything I was told. I lay still. I tried to control the moans that frequently escaped my lips, to be silent, to not be a nuisance. My jaw hurt from clenching, but there was nothing either of us could do to convince anyone just how excruciating my body felt as it struggled against wave after wave of pain. Desperate to help, Neil ended up phoning our GP to see if there was anything he could do to intervene. I don't think anyone in the Emergency Department appreciated his 'interference.' I began to realise just how isolated chronic pain sufferers are and how inadequately emergency departments are prepped for dealing with this condition. It isn't acknowledged as a genuine condition. They didn't know us before 'the pain' and, while we might not be a life-and-death risk, we are in a terrible state.

Chronic pain is a whole-body experience that is unexplainable. Doctors typically ask you to rate that pain level out of 10, or to be specific as to how it feels and where it is. The pain monster is far too invasive and much cleverer than that! The medical staff get unsettled by this elusive condition.

They had no idea what I was feeling or why I wasn't improving. Each time they touched me, I screamed involuntarily. I couldn't help it. My skin felt like it was on fire. Every movement caused unbearable pain throughout my back, my chest, everywhere. I desperately needed to use the toilet, but it was impossible to get a bed pan under me. I ended up wetting the bed. It was humiliating and painful when they took the soiled sheets away for disposal. I had no dignity left. I had no care. I just wanted it all to stop. It seemed that no one treating me understood what I was going through, probably because they had never themselves had to live with chronic pain for every second of every minute of every hour of every day of their life. A single tear escaped once more and slid slowly down my already tear-stained cheek. I closed my eyes and gritted my teeth, praying for that darkness to envelop me once more. And Neil, poor Neil, felt helpless by my side, until his advocacy kicked in.

Unable to get back into the hospital I had so often attended over the past few years, where I felt safe and knew the staff, we were desperate for some direction. Neil insisted that the staff in the Emergency Department called other facilities to find me a space. Finally, they found a vacancy at a hospital 40 minutes away. Thank goodness I had Neil there, fighting my fight. I have no idea what I would have done without him. Having found the bed, he then had to plead with the staff to organise the transfer as soon as possible. Don't get me wrong, I understand that Emergency Departments are for emergencies, and priority of course must always be given to saving lives. But I had been there, as one day merged into the next, like a forgotten shadow except for the cries and screams which involuntarily leaped unfettered from my throat, reminding the staff I was still in the corridor! I was in desperate pain and they couldn't fix it-but there was a distinct lack of understanding of the genuine discomfort Neil and I were in as we tried to cope with the situation. Two hours later, in the early hours of the morning, I was on the move again. I was terrified, going into yet another facility, people I didn't know and having to try and explain the unexplainable yet again.

Having taken prescription opioids for so long, I was constantly not only forgetting things, but I was repeating myself and vehemently denying that I had been told something just a few moments or a day or so earlier. It was frustrating and caused tension. My sense of self altered. I became lost and cranky. Sometimes I would be OK, thinking I was back to my old self, then the darkness and confusion would roll in like a clap of thunder, causing the storm in my brain which altered the moment, that day and those years. I didn't know that I was poisoning myself, making everything worse. Obviously, my caring GP didn't either. Only now do we know that long-term opioid use is a recipe for disaster; for many, death. I didn't escape those thoughts. Many times, I wanted to die, to not continue in this trapped mind and body anymore. Well, maybe I didn't want to die, but I had no other means of escaping this nightmare; to dispose of the confusion, the lost me that with each passing day was getting more and more away from my sense of who I was, my connection with myself and the world around me. How easy to die, how difficult to live! My thoughts were scattered, my mind was dulled, and my pain was sharp.

But alternate pathways were limited, in terms of knowledge, geographic and financial reach. I needed something to manage the pain, yet I wasn't comprehending that my pain wasn't being managed. More of the same drugs, more of the same reaction. A constant state of chronic pain with intermittent acute episodes led to months out of action, brain drain, fatigue and despair. Not to mention the constipation and nausea from the concoction of medications. And all that puts pressure on the back, adding yet another layer to this complex situation. It was getting worse, not better.

At one stage, in yet another hospital 'stay', the neuropathy was frustrating and the treatment I was receiving was doing nothing to alleviate my agony. I was sent to a Brisbane hospital in an attempt to uncover what was causing the pain and my inability to stand without dropping to the floor in pain.

Despite being under a renowned neurologist, I had yet another awful medication-related experience which interestingly, I recall with clarity. Funny how the brain does that!

I had been given Lyrica, a common drug for neuropathic pain. I'm tall and slim, perhaps a little underweight as, for me, food wasn't of interest when my pain was fierce. But my low weight shouldn't be relevant, as drug dosages are matched with weight and medical history. My dose of Lyrica had been increased the day before to 100mg, still on the low side, but remember I am allergic to morphine, sensitive to other drugs and prone to fits following anaesthetic. So, enough history to be cautious, one would like to think. This afternoon I was experiencing some strange sensations and reported them to the nurses. I was sensing fireworks in my head, an unusual body sensation and I felt 'most odd'. This is where the sense of not being believed or equally as frustrating, catastrophising, played itself out. I remember it was 2.15pm and I called the nurse, explaining how I felt. Rather off-handily, she said to just lay down and relax, it will pass. I was scared and knew this wasn't normal, but obviously was unable to emphasise my predicament sufficiently to be believed. I was exhausted from the pain, two-and-a-half hours from home and feeling vulnerable. The sensations got worse and I discovered that I couldn't move my left arm to press the buzzer for help. My left side started to drop, and I could feel I was drooling. But I was stuck. Terrified, I lay there, my mind exploding with fear, trapped in this useless body. I can't explain the feeling, except to say, if I thought I was scared before, this was a whole new level. At 5.15pm, what I can only explain as a miracle happened.

Shae is a nurse and was working in Brisbane at the time. She came in to see me after work and, with one look, hit the emergency button. By this stage I was terrified. As far as I was aware, no one had been in to check on me even though I had previously implored that something wasn't right. I had spent the last three hours terrified, trapped, unable to move, and I had lost my ability to speak. Drool was falling out of the left side of my mouth and the features on my face had dropped. Later we were told that a nurse had 'popped her head round' but thought I was asleep. For heaven's sake, I was stuck in my body!

Lights flashed; people talked loudly. A sense of urgency as you see in the movies when someone has a heart attack, started to play out all around me. I could hear what everyone was saying, but I was unable to respond. I know they called my family to come immediately, unsure what was happening but treating it as serious. Neil made the two-hour trip in record time. My poor family had been given the fright of their lives, unsure if I was going to survive this incident. The outcome was, thankfully, an unusual reaction to the medication which caused this stroke-like condition. I was 'back to normal' within 48 hours, but I have never forgotten the horrendous experience. I'm not sure what was worse, being able to hear but not communicate or move, or the fact that no one believed me, no one validated the sensations I was experiencing. It was another example of this nonspecific chronic pain condition being so misunderstood, and the frustration of the too-often accusations of catastrophising.

It wasn't all bad. I had some very supportive hospital stays, with caring staff and pain and rehabilitation programs attached to the hospital. There were many occasions when I felt safe in the hospital, cared for, and that I was making good progress. But sadly, progress was always short-lived, and the frustrations of a day in the life of an unwilling member of the pain tribe continued.

I had attended pain programs, and found they had both positive and negative impacts for me. At one of the outpatient programs I attended, I did get a better understanding of what pain is and a little about the relationship between pain, thoughts and physical activity. The exercises were good when I was able to participate, and the comradery of being with people in similar circumstances was certainly a plus. In fact, I am still in contact with one of the participants. She and I have an understanding and just 'get it' when we share our frustrations. Equally, we share in the good times and try to raise each other up when life gets tricky. I also continue to see the physiotherapist who presented at the pain program; she has been a major part of my healing process. I felt less isolated and a little more understood. The downside was that once the program was finished and flare-ups happened again, I would feel a sense of failure and lack of hope. That 'here we go again' scenario played in my head. Yes, I was able to put some of the strategies I had learnt into practice, but I was still heavily medicated, and my general mood was low. I needed some ongoing support and I didn't know where else to find it.

At times I was unable to speak, to function in society or at home. My world had become so small, so suffocating, I needed to find a way out. But I was lost. Neil and I needed to find something new, but where to look? We had tried so many avenues, but they were limited by location and existing knowledge. I was stuck, going through endless revolving doors of hope and shattering letdown, searching for answers and finding none. Many specialists had an opinion of a possible 'cure', only to be countered by other specialists with opposing views. I decided enough was enough. No more specialists, no more invasive surgeries. I had to find another way.

## Light amidst the darkness

I mentioned before that after two days in the Emergency Department, I was sent to a hospital that I hadn't previously attended. It was confronting and I admit to feeling scared, having to explain the unexplainable all over again – and face what I felt was the stigma of chronic pain. I am a woman of integrity, of truth, not prone to exaggeration. I am not one that enjoys attention, particularly when it's all negative. Unfortunately, the medical staff didn't know the 'then me' – they only knew the 'now me', the 'pain me'; my experience over these past difficult years was that they couldn't see the person behind the pain. I was now carrying this defensive suit of armour; this need to be believed yet unable to find a way to make that happen.

But all this changed over the next ten weeks.

> After a few weeks in hospital, getting gradual relief from my pain, I was seen by a pain specialist from the rehabilitation unit. I was clearly not yet ready to go home, having major difficulty in moving to a standing position and walking to the bathroom. It was suggested that I move to the rehabilitation unit where I would be supported by a team of specialists. I was still feeling low, desperate to be rid of my life as it was, out of control and

sad. To be honest, I didn't have much choice. I couldn't stay where I was, and I couldn't go home. So, I was moved, painfully yet with care, to the rehabilitation unit where I was settled into my own room even though it was a public facility. That was a bonus in one way, but the other side of the coin is that distraction is an excellent therapy. Not having someone to talk to, I thought I might get even lower in my despair. I was feeling very much on the edge.

It was 11am on a Thursday when my life changed. I was told that a physiotherapist would come in and talk to me. My immediate thought was: 'Here we go again, total lack of understanding. How on earth can I engage in physiotherapy when every movement hurts so much?'

Boy, was I wrong! And this is a good example of the importance of not generalising. Not all physiotherapists treat with the same techniques, not all people over 70 need the same support, not all dogs bite – you get my drift? Sharon sat next to me and held my hand. Yes, it's true.

She sat quietly, calmly, and asked me: 'What do you want, Dawn? What do you need?'

'I want to die,' I replied.

We sat together. The tears flowed freely for the first time in a very long time. I was being heard, I was being treated as a human being, not a member of the catastrophising pain tribe. Someone was asking me what I needed, not telling me what I need to do, what should work, and then never does.

I remember I was emotionally exhausted for the rest of that day. Still practically bed bound, I felt a massive release as a combination of emotional and physical fatigue overwhelmed my whole being. Sharon 'got it', she seemed to understand my despair and, more importantly, understand that this was real, the pain was horrendous, and I was stuck.

My mind, body and soul had become stuck in this world of pain, protecting itself and, in so doing, creating a life on the run, forever ducking and weaving (metaphorically speaking) from the next pain onslaught. And not only the pain onslaught, the lack of answers, the absence of any protection for this ongoing, debilitating, life-sapping dis-ease.

Over the next ten weeks I was fortunate enough to be part of a residential rehabilitation program headed up by a pain specialist who was trained in Europe. She was the first person to offer some explanation of my pain that made sense, which matched what was happening to me. She recognised that it was real and needed a holistic approach to management. And she had a pathway for that approach. Hallelujah!

During that time in rehabilitation, I had my ups and downs, working with some therapists who didn't seem to understand but, in the main, it was positive. Sharon was my guide, my saving grace, and I continued to work with her at an external pain program a few months after my release. The main difference was she wasn't offering an either/or, nor was she suggesting a quick fix. Sharon approached my pain as a mind, body, soul integrated condition, and while I wasn't aware of it at the time, she prepared my pathway to a whole new way of managing my disability.

Because it was a disability, it still is a disability. But unlike many other disabilities or chronic conditions which are physically obvious and socially accepted, chronic pain can be obvious sometimes and hidden at other times. So, people think you are 'better', 'healed', 'fixed'. Hell, I even go down that track sometimes. But the reality is that it's always there, and the key to living a life that has joy, laughter, friendships and passion is learning to manage that disability. To own it and to work with it, not against it. To accept that it is there but, over time, it can offer benefits you never ever imagined. If someone had said that to me a year or two ago, I would have gladly stuck a dagger in their eye, believing they had no idea what I was going through. Well now, maybe they don't know what I am going through, but I do, at least I have a better appreciation of it, and that's what matters.

# Reflections from this Chapter

- Pain has a flow on effect to everyone around us. This means that support needs to be extended to the family unit, not just the individual who is experiencing the pain.
- Pain impacts our relationships; we are confused, fearful, have smashed dreams, often terrified of the change, often live with self-doubt and experience frustrating brain fog.
- There is so much stigma attached to NDRCP, both internal and external. It's important to smash this perception and educate health professionals and the wider public on the challenges of living with NDRCP.
- Many NDRCP sufferers live with heavy guilt.

- Pain and fear are inevitable bedfellows fear of the pain, fear of the shame and fear of the future.
- Grief is a significant aspect of pain – life as we knew it, gone. But if we shift our understanding of pain, we can learn to rebuild our lives and use our experiences in a positive way.
- Pain is exhausting, physically, emotionally, mentally and spiritually. So we need to adjust our life accordingly.
- Pain signals are real, long after there is a real pain threat. To understand this principle, we need to hear it from someone we trust.
- Pacing is a life skill that's difficult to learn – especially when you have those wonderful moments of energy.
- Some hospital experiences are great; others unfortunately, contribute to our sense of despair.
- Emergency Departments have a long way to go to improve understanding and support for NDRCP patients.
- Sometimes, things happen unexpectedly. Finding Sharon was

the beginning of my path to recovery.

# Part Three

# Finding a Path to Acceptance

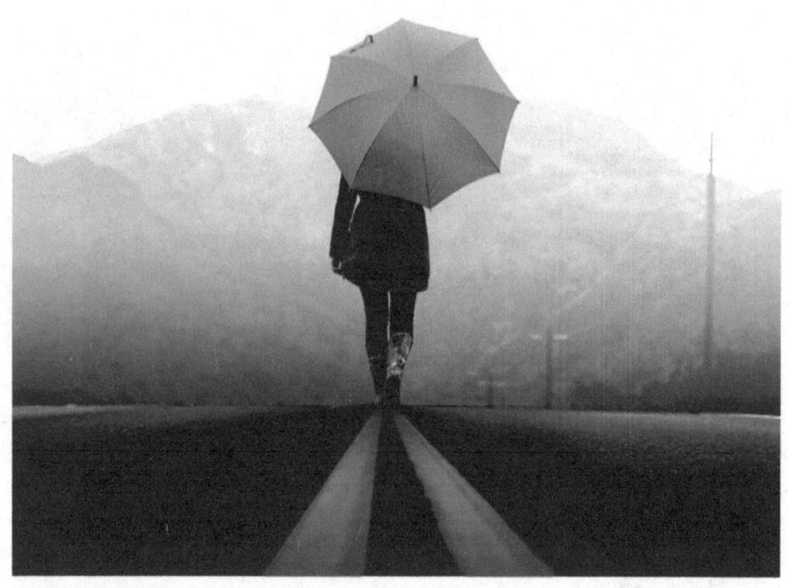

# 9

# I'M BEGINNING TO UNDERSTAND

***If one is master of one thing and understands one thing well, one has at the same time, insight into and understanding of many things.***
**Vincent Van Gogh**

A lot of people have asked me what I did to 'get better'. That question stumped me for a while because there wasn't any particular moment, no magic bullet. Or at least I thought there wasn't. Oh, and by the way, I'm not 'better'. But I am definitely managing my pain better. Most of the time!

Certainly, the fact that my 'condition' was real and validated was a major turning point, and my continued work with Sharon helped me understand how pain actually invades our body and our mind; how our muscles and our cells hold memories that may no longer be useful in the current situation. I now know what 'it's all in your head' actually means. Used correctly, sensitively and in context, it's not a derogatory statement, but a fact. Our brains receive messages via the spinal cord, which is the tunnel, the gateway for sensory signals. The brain regulates how much pain we feel in two main ways. There can be an increase in inflammation messages via a chemical reaction which is called neurogenic information, and the pathways that filter pain start to degrade if pain is experienced for more than three to four weeks. After that, the brain becomes overly plastic, affecting the functional connectivity and the accuracy of the neurogenic information, the pain message.

In my case, I experienced both nociceptive pain and neuropathic pain. Put simply, the former is due to actual spinal damage and arthritis, the latter is damage to the nerves. In other words, neuropathic pain is pain caused by changes in the central nervous system which occur long after the physical damage is healed and is a major cause of my chronic pain. Even when there is no new physical damage, my central nervous system responds to my thoughts and the environment, becomes excited and sends messages to my brain that are interpreted as pain. And it is therefore real. This is often referred to as Central Nervous System Sensitisation.

So, understanding this, the logic was to do something about these pain messages. But how?

Even though I had been told this, I didn't know what to do with the information as I was always so exhausted, had so much brain fog that going down any new, exploratory path was too much of an effort for my fuzzy brain to handle. My short-term memory was terrible, often swearing blind that something hadn't happened, or someone hadn't said what they were adamant they had told me. It was like seeing a faint light in the distance, a beckoning glow at the end of a dangerous tunnel full of unknown spaces, out of reach, yet my only hope. But I had been disappointed so many times before by suggestions of how to cure my condition, I admit that I was close to feeling defeated, to not believing, not trusting, yet I had this tension between defeat, accepting my diminished pain-stricken, restricted life, or trying to muster the energy to keep trying.

The other side of this was that even though it was logical, I still couldn't get rid of the sense it was a bit hocus pocus, a bit of a placebo approach, and therefore that stigma about the pain not being 'real' hung over me like a dark shadow. You may recall I am psychology-trained, have worked as a clinician for 30 years, so whilst the emphasis on the mind was a comfortable space for me to hold, the connection between mind, body and soul was a bit 'out there'. I now find that a scary thought and am embarrassed that through all those years of practice, I wasn't clear enough about that connection. But the reality is, there are psychologists and other therapists who continue to practice in a silo, focussing only on their specific modality, totally dismissing the essential connection between mind, body and soul.

***

17 August 2017 is a day etched in my brain forever. It was both the end, and a beginning. The day I finally weaned myself off all the opioids I had been on for three years. I wasn't getting any better and, having attended all the 'services' suggested by my GP, and the pain programs, the only solution I was left with was to take even more drugs. But nothing was changing – I was still in a world of hurt, a world of pain and a micro world of fuzzy memory, inability to form proper sentences or hold a decent conversation.

So somehow, somewhere in my brain I decided to come off the medication and, even though I did it gradually, I imagine it was like coming down from heroin. I didn't know what to expect, as I hadn't been a drug addict before the pain had taken over my life. I don't honestly think I believed the prescribed medications I was taking could be so damaging. But there I was, itchy skin, even worse night's sleep than before, this time accompanied by hot and cold sweats which were not menopause (I was on HRT), anxiety through the roof and edgy all the time. But on 17 August 2017, I started to feel better. I felt a clarity in my mind, a fog lifting and, excuse the pun, a new dawn approaching.

From that moment, I could start to take control of my pain. That meant I could start to get some control of my life back. And this is what I discovered I needed when my brain started to un-fog:

- ongoing support
- to shift my thinking, change my communication style and stop apologising for my condition
- to change my habits – keep the good, dump the bad (that doesn't mean no wine or chocolate by the way) and create new ones
- to stop protecting my pain
- to dump all my negative labels, the words that described how useless I was, and replace them with authentic, positive labels
- to change my social environment
- to push myself when I felt I couldn't cope (learning to pace)
- to stop pushing myself (learning not to race)

- to make changes to my physical environment
- to learn more about the mind/body/soul connection
- to find a way to quieten my central nervous system, to minimise those pain messages
- to activate my parasympathetic nervous system
- to accept that I was never going to be the 'then Dawn'
- to embrace the 'now Dawn'
- to acknowledge that, in accepting this change, there is grief and loss to be worked through
- to 'sit with it', to be present in whatever state I was in at the time
- to acknowledge that there will be flare-ups
- to find joy again
- to be a mother, a grandma and a wife again
- to live for each day, yet have a plan for the future
- to find a passion, a reason to live
- to be trusted and respected for my choices
- to trust myself

- to find a way of contributing to society
- to let others know about my journey so they could talk more about this 'silent epidemic' and support all those affected by this chronic disease

As a health professional and educator, I realised I needed to take action so that medical and allied health professions learn to be more understanding of the impact they have with their language and their tone. I also want health professionals to support the exploration of complimentary pathways to enhance the management of chronic pain. This is my responsibility – and this book is one of the ways I plan to continue and execute all the above.

In the words of Mahatma Gandhi, I need to:

*Be the change that you wish to see in the world.*

In this case, the word 'be' is a verb, I had to posit a shift in my current 'be'ing, and the world was my world. I needed to do it, but it didn't mean I had to do it alone.

I notice I have written most of the above in the past tense, a realisation of what was missing perhaps and what has now become clear. I won't rewrite the list in the present tense, but I invite you to read it in both the present and the past tense, because this is an ongoing challenge. Some days some of these things are a breeze because they have become an integral part of the new me, other days, it's hard. But I will keep on keeping on – because it matters, I matter.

Knowing what we need, and actually getting what we need, can be quite different. In sharing some of my experiences, I thought perhaps it would clarify some of the challenges as well as some of the positive outcomes that living in this world of pain has presented.

## Ongoing Support

As humans, we have not evolved to live in isolation and hence we offer support to each other in many different ways. As a chronic pain sufferer, or carer of someone with chronic pain, we need to find support beyond what may appear obvious, or available. It's interesting, that the experience of Covid-19 has offered the global population an insight into living with fear and isolation. I have spoken to many people over these past few months who tell me that suddenly, the isolation of living with chronic pain feels less than before. Isolation is often accompanied by fear, and seen as a stigmatised way to live, yet during COVID-19, it became the new norm. This has connected many chronic pain sufferers to the outside world in a way they never could have imagined, primarily, and interestingly, helping them feel less alone.

## Medical

I recognise that I needed support from the medical profession, to be treated as whole person, not just focussing on the symptoms. I certainly had wonderful professional, skilled support in spades for other medical issues, and skilled surgeons to whom I am forever grateful. But when it came to managing my chronic pain, that support was not only limited, with all the best of intentions, I believe that for much of the time, it was doing me more harm than good.

It's a tough one. I needed diagnosis to try and help me understand and treat my condition. That was part of the problem. In the past 5 years, it's become evident that chronic pain is often difficult to diagnose and even harder to treat or manage, specifically NDRCP. Each doctor or specialist seemed to be searching for a one-off cause and I was left with a confusion of what was actually wrong with me. I now realise it doesn't matter because the way in which I manage my multiple conditions is the same, irrespective of the number of labels I put on it. And it's even more complicated if you have insurance companies involved and/or needing financial support as was my situation. However, although I had to jump through many hoops and opinions, and exhausting, confronting and emotionally draining appointments before having my insurance activated, I am forever grateful for that support.

My GP was great, but unfortunately I think he was stuck in the medical model, so medication was his main 'go to', which ultimately became my biggest challenge to overcome. To be fair, he did suggest I see a psychologist (which I was actually pretty pissed off about because I read that to mean it was all in my head – and you know the old interpretation of that saying) but my experience with the particular person I was referred to was less than satisfactory. And perhaps if he himself had understood the mechanics of chronic pain, he would have been able to explain to me why I needed to find a range of strategies to help me live with this condition. But two things are apparent here; the first is that chronic pain is only just being recognised 'as a condition' and the second, is that GP's are not educated in the complexity of chronic pain and therefore it was beyond his scope of understanding to know what else to suggest. Added to that, it seems that GP's do not have a list of counsellors or psychologists who specialise in chronic pain – this needs to be addressed (I'll get to that later).

Not having one diagnosis is tricky, but often, like in my case, what was actually wrong with me was never discussed, or at least if it was, I don't remember. In fact, the only validation from a medical person was a wonderful doctor I saw in the rehabilitation unit. Even then, there were no labels, just an acknowledgement that the pain was real, it was complicated and there is no one specific answer. But what I have learnt is that when there is no further bone damage yet the brain is still telling me I am in pain, most doctors seem to throw their hands up. No obvious damage showing in X-rays or MRI's = no pain.

WRONG!

Pain specialists now know that's not the case and that the alarm system in our brain is triggered legitimately and creates pain. But not having this explained and having to wait to discover this far later along my dehumanising pain journey, is what I consider to be a travesty of justice. Still, I get it now, and recognise that I am not being a hypochondriac or going insane when I say that my mood affects my pain, because there is a chemical and neurological link to these actions.

Having said that, it's important to remember that every person living with chronic pain has a different lived experience based on the years leading up to 'today'. In my case, it's not only mood or cognitive activity which impacts on my pain. Multiple surgeries, hospital and decades of pain experiences have left my body with limited muscle strength which in turn creates ongoing difficulties in establishing pain free moments.

## Family and Friends

Family is what's most important to me and therefore the most significant piece to this complex puzzle. Neil's unswerving love and support is what's made these past years manageable, rich and meaningful. He was, and is, my rock, yet we still found ourselves creating distance and emotional shut down as we navigated this cruel path. Probably the most important part of his support was his advocacy for my wellbeing. He was my voice when I couldn't speak, my nurse when I couldn't move and my best friend when I felt bereft. He handled all the hospital things when I was totally incapable of making any decisions. He was by my side at all times, though I must admit, that in itself was sometimes too much, and we had to talk about that too. Because I felt such a burden, on many occasions I wanted my space, not to feel that he felt he had to be by my side. I wanted him to go and have a life outside of my pain and, by him not doing that, I often felt an even greater burden. Gradually, we have learnt to recognise each other's needs through improved language and communication. Until recently, it was not so easy with my children. I struggled with telling them too much, with saying I'm OK when I'm not. The worst thing was when they would ask: 'And what are you doing today?'

And up until the latter part of 2019, my answer was often so flipping boring, so empty. Gone were the days when I could share with them a fun, packed schedule of discovery and learning. However, it's definitely getting better, although I am acutely aware of the relatively sedentary life, I now lead compared to what my life was. I now have a lovely social life and arrange times to catch up with friends, go to the movies and enjoy meals together. The more my pain is under control, the more my interests expand and the more interesting my conversations. In January 2020 I returned again to the UK and had a wonderful time with family and friends. No great flare-ups, and I was careful to pace, not race.

That being said since gaining a better understanding of chronic pain management, and having years of rest to reclaim my body and appreciate the direct connection between mind, body and soul, now, in 2020, I am amazed at where I am.

Apart from the sense of achievement in writing this book, I have rebuilt my counselling practice across an international platform. Neil has built me a home office and I mainly work from home, so I am not adding pressure on my body by getting in and out the car more often than necessary. I 'see' clients via phone, zoom or many of the virtual platforms now available to us. Through the COVID-19 pandemic, I feel honoured to be amongst the thousands of frontline workers offering my support at times of significant anxiety and global disruption. I often refer to my pain experience when supporting people through difficult times, sharing the importance of building resilience, practising self-compassion and identifying relevant supports. I have also delivered training programs on building resilience and effective communication and was proud to be invited as a keynote speaker to share my story of resilience and hope to an audience of 200 education professionals.

Although, here is an honest peep into the time leading up to that talk, not shared with anyone until now. My pain was heightened, and I knew I had to work hard on controlling my fear. I told myself constantly to focus on the 'what is' and not the 'what if', an essential strategy for dealing with anxiety and fear. Nonetheless, it was a frustrating battle. Neil had to come with me to the conference as my support, both to drive me there and as my rock 'in case' anything happened.

I was to speak on day two – and I managed to circulate with conference delegates on the first day. I was aware of the pressure building up and the expectation to deliver to a prestigious audience. That night in the hotel room, I couldn't get rid of an excruciating head and neck ache, and my back was causing me real concerns. Stabbing pains kept trying to bring me down, taking me back to the Dawn I had hoped was less present. By 3am, I hadn't slept a wink and was constantly getting up to cope with the nausea. Thank goodness Neil was with me. At 6am he scoured the local area and found a chemist for anti-nausea tablets. I always have pain killers with me but hadn't thought about that one! Note to self for next time (because there will be another keynote, another conference, and I will be more prepared).

As they say, the show must go on. I dressed, paced around the room, walked out into the fresh air and had no idea how I was going to pull this off. Somehow, I got to the lectern and organised everything, so I didn't have to look down, because tilting my head down to read anything caused waves of sickness and blurred vision. I had a chair placed up on the stage too, in case I needed to sit because of the pain.

But you know, I did it! I focussed on my story and the topic of the day, building hope and resilience. I was proud of my presentation and even more proud of the fact that I don't think anyone had a clue about my struggle that day. Until now. And, because I managed to deliver, 200 people now know some of the challenges we have when we live with chronic pain, and how so many of those challenges help build strength and courage, and how when our worlds change, we can still find a way through. So now I have something to talk about.

During the really dark times, and when these frightening experiences come back to haunt me, reminding me that I am fragile and always in a management phase, that it's not going to 'go away'. I realised that there was no one I could talk to about the impact of my pain, apart from Neil. I hadn't been able to find a good psychologist or counsellor with an understanding of my lived concerns. I am not saying there aren't some out there, but finding them is the challenge. And sometimes the burden of all these mixed emotions, of feeling lost, scared, uncertain, a burden etc., etc. weighed heavy. I now understand that when our emotions are awry, this too can send my sympathetic nervous system into overload and cause more pain signals, followed by the inevitable cycle of flare-ups. So, trying to manage my emotions, express my feelings but not get stuck in the misery of them, is an important part of managing my pain.

Friends were great – always checking in and, importantly, supporting Neil when I was in hospital. However, this was a double-edged sword as whilst it was good to stay connected, I felt very disconnected from everyone, always wearing a mask and saying I was better than I was because how I felt was so boring and so there was little authenticity in our conversations. I felt this new Dawn had nothing of value to contribute, so even when I was energised enough to have a conversation, often it left me feeling empty. And one of the hardest things is when well-meaning friends ask: 'And what exactly is wrong with your back?'

This is such a difficult question, as the answer is too complicated and, to be honest, I don't think they really want the details. It's often to compare with themselves or someone else they know who has had 'the same'. The conversation often went like this along the lines of: 'This treatment worked really well for "XYZ"—they are fine now.'

Leaving me feeling yet again that I am not trying hard enough to resolve my pain. All that being said, please stick with it. I am now so grateful to all those people who stayed with us and didn't give up just because I was 'less than' for so many years. THANK YOU.

## I needed to shift my thinking and my language

This one is simple, but hard to apply. I needed to stop thinking of my situation as a disaster, ruining my life and impeding my every move, shrinking my life to a tiny geographic and intellectual zone. To a life bereft of touch (because it hurt so much), disconnected from those I love in the real, authentic sense of me. I needed to believe again, to trust I could manage this and that I was in charge of my own destiny. The medical profession use this awful word, 'catastrophising', and when they say that, I get an acute sense of being judged, of the realisation that they had no idea of the effect this debilitating pain has on my life. It's a word that should be used with a greater degree of care and context, but looking back now, that's what I was doing. And our words are so powerful. Our thoughts affect our feelings, our feelings affect our thoughts. And words are one way of expressing these thoughts and feelings. Although, at times, the pain IS catastrophic!

When I was so heavily medicated, none of this was possible; but once off all the opioids, I was able to see opportunities for alternate pathways, for other ways to manage my life. That was because:

- my pain was no worse without the medication (although I was really nervous about not having the medications as a crutch, a backup)
- I realised I had lost chunks of memory and had difficulty finding words although my memory is still affected, this has improved considerably over time
- my thinking was clearer once off the meds
- my speech was more articulate and more interesting (at last)
- I needed to take control and not give away my power ever again
- I started to seek ways to calm my nervous system, to alter the messages to my brain, because I recognised that was the missing piece of my puzzle.

## Language

Once I realised this, Neil and I worked together on my language – and his. I had to encourage him not to mollycoddle me, not to try and do everything for me. It was making me feel incapable, over-reliant and helpless. I told him that I would ask if I needed anything and to please stop asking if I was OK. I wanted our conversations to be different, to not always be focussed around my pain. It has been difficult for him to adapt; it's an ongoing process, but we are doing well.

Of course, that meant I had to admit to when I was struggling, though it was usually etched all over my face. It's strange: this condition (although still not officially accepted as a 'condition', which is a whole other argument) is referred to as the invisible or silent disease, yet I know that the expressions on my face, the exhausted lines around my eyes and the pallor of my skin told its own story to those that knew me. We are always aware of our communication style and we are often reminding each other about what works best for us – but it's truly worth doing. The benefits include helping me feel that I am a partner, not a child in need of help. It makes me feel more in charge of myself, more equal in the relationship.

A good example of my compromise is hanging out the washing. On good days I will ask Neil to carry the basket to the washing line and I will hang the washing out. He no longer tries to do it all, recognising, because I have articulated it many times, that I can stretch, and that this movement is good for me. And it means he isn't doing everything. The same with the cleaning. I do what I can, usually at standing level, like washing up, wiping the benchtops and the blinds. I'm not stupid enough to try and tuck in the corners of sheets or vacuum – but I am doing my share and that matters to me.

On the flip side, I am learning to say when I am having a rough patch and need to take things slow. That's a real contrast to the 'then Dawn', when I did a million things at once and always operated on high energy levels. I still find that admission of pain and exhaustion challenging because it is such a contrast, but I know that if I self-care, I won't end up back in hospital, relying on a medical answer when there is none, or certainly none that I would entertain. I give myself permission to slow down – and that's truly a new thing for me.

## Dumping bad habits and creating new ones

The first thing I needed to realise was which habits were inhibiting my pain management and which habits were helping. This was an interesting exercise. I was very protective of my learnt pain-protection habits, so I often went into defence mode and justified to myself why I was acting or thinking that way. It's hard to be objective about this, because I was so invested in protecting myself from the pain, I thought I was doing everything I could to make that happen. This is where a chronic pain counsellor would have been so useful – but I couldn't find one.

## Protecting my pain

One thing I reluctantly realised, was that in protecting my pain, I was causing more pain. I say 'reluctantly' because I was sure I was doing everything I could NOT to be in pain and induce flare-ups. I now recognise that at times, I was doing exactly the opposite! Whenever I felt that knife serrating its way through my back, or the flying bullets down my leg, I would brace and immediately my thoughts would go to: *Oh no, here we go again. Please, please, no!* And with that, my body would stiffen, a heaviness would engulf me, and I felt defeated, anticipating what was to come next. So, with Neil's help, we created a few sentences that changed my thinking:

*This is only a single message, not a disaster.*

*Take a few gentle breaths focusing on each inhale and exhale.*

*Decide for myself—shall I keep moving gently or is it best to lie down for a while?*

Over this past year or so, I have really noticed the benefits of this self-talk. If I relax into the pain rather than stiffen up, my body is less likely to spasm as I am not creating a trigger effect. It's a bit like if you are caught in a rip; the advice is to swim across it, not against it. Going against anything is exhausting, a drain on the mind because of the stress, and similarly on the body. So, it makes sense to be in the moment, and without a doubt, it is proving to make a big difference.

## Social life

Other bad habits that needed a swift kick out the door included not shying away from making social arrangements. I became brave and told my friends that I would love to plan something together, but if I was unable to make it, I hope they would understand. That was a BIG step for me, as I hated to admit that I was struggling, yet of course, everyone was well aware! The other big plus in making this change was recognising the importance of divergence therapy, taking my mind off the pain and frustration and getting involved in something I enjoy.

In my early 20s when I was living in London, I worked for a short stint as a Play Therapist at St Bartholomew's Hospital. I have always known the benefits of taking one's mind off whatever is troubling you, even if it's a temporary reprieve; yet applying that to myself when I was in my brain fog and acute pain just didn't happen. Of course, the other significant issue is that when you are in excruciating pain, if someone tells you to think of something else, you just want to murder them. It seems like an impossible request and highlights yet again that no one is even close to understanding how awful the pain is and that it's not my choice to be in that pain moment. But having created the time and space to review this, I see the benefits. And it's all about benefits; about what can make that particular moment more manageable.

It was difficult for Neil at times, because I would insist that I was OK to go out or sometimes invite people here even if I was in a real pickle. I wanted to believe that I could handle it; at least it was better to have the pain and some fun, rather than just be home and have only the pain to focus on. Yes, there were times when that didn't work out so well, but the more I put myself out there, the more confident I became and the more I was able to achieve some semblance of social life.

And the internal stigma I was carrying was just that – internal. It was a label, a habit I had developed, assuming people would get sick of me because of my frequent bailing out of events due to pain, or if I did manage to be present, I wasn't exactly a bundle of fun, the 'Then Dawn' being lost and the 'Now Dawn' struggling to be good company. I thought they would stop wanting me as part of their lives. I now know that was the farthest thing from the truth. However, if numbers were an issue, or a financial commitment before the event such as tickets for a show, well, I am only just beginning to go there. However, I was, and still am to some degree, sensitive to the knowledge that I can't be relied on for important engagements because one of my biggest frustrations (I know, there have been many) is the unpredictability of my pain. I can literally be getting into the car, or maybe arrived at my destination, and as I put another foot forward, bang! In those circumstances, it just is what it is. I must accept that, and it's a hard lesson, acknowledging that they were being realistic about my ability to commit to something that impacted others. The 'Then Dawn' was always reliable, determined to always follow through; that has been one of the hardest adjustments to make. But it's OK (most of the time), because I now have a far more realistic perspective of what I can and can't do. And whereas in the four years when my pain was in total control of me, the odds were 95% unlikely to complete an engagement Now, it's more like 90% likely that I can show up, and I'm pretty happy with that.

## Learning to pace, not race

Probably my biggest challenge I can blame on my A type personality, and the fact that I am a Capricorn. It's often good to have something else to blame! I have always been a busy person, and my idea of busy seems to be far busier, more hectic, than many of my friends. The flip side of that is my idea of pacing, not racing, (in other words, slowing down), doesn't seem to be particularly slow to many people. All of us members of the pain tribe know that a fundamental part of our pain management is to 'pace, not race', a term we are probably all sick of hearing. It's a basic tool for pain management but incredibly difficult once you have some energy back, some clarity of mind. Because what accompanies that returned energy and clarity is the want to 'do'. And for me, the 'doing' was always 'all or nothing', going hammer and tongs until what I had set my mind to do was completed.

I have learnt the hard way. I still set goals – writing this book, for instance – but my goals are now far more realistic, and I always (well, most of the time), factor in a rest in-between. I also know that I cannot juggle as many things in one day, or one week for that matter, as I did before in my old life. But that's OK, I accept that again, most of the time!

# Changes to my physical environment

Physically there were (and still are) occasions when I needed assistance. When the pain was excruciating, I used a modified toilet seat which raised the height. Yes, I still screamed as I tried to lower myself down, but at least there wasn't quite so far to go, and with the help of Neil and the arms of the seat, I could at least use a toilet, most of the time. I also have a shower chair on hand, aids to pick things up from the floor, shoehorns and yes, my sky-blue walking stick, all invaluable aids. The twist to having these aids is it puts fairly and squarely in your face that you are disabled. And that, as you probably already know, is seriously confronting.

On one occasion, the rehabilitation unit organised for an occupational therapist to come to our home and assess what could be adapted to make my life easier. It was a wonderful service. They organised an additional step for the front door, discussed changes in our bathroom, and supplied a more appropriate chair for when I could sit for a period of time and watch television or read; but in the main, they were happy with the design of our home. I suppose that's no surprise, as we did purpose-build our home and, as my back has been a challenge for so long, we specifically designed it as single-level with higher-than-usual bench tops (I'm quite tall) and large doorways to accommodate a wheelchair. Whilst I haven't used a wheelchair in the home, as Neil is often supporting me through a doorway to the bedroom (not what you are thinking!), the extra width has been useful as two, sometimes three bodies try to navigate the space supporting me. One adaptation I have made is the positioning of the toilet roll. I found that the slight twist to the side was often enough to send my back into spasm. So, the toilet roll is now positioned slightly in front of the toilet to minimise stretching and twisting.

I had to sell my car for four reasons. I wasn't able to drive, (I guess that's as good a reason as any), it was too low for me to get in and out of, the doors were heavy (it was a two-seater sports), and as I wasn't working and Neil was my unofficial carer, we couldn't afford to keep two cars. We bought an old Toyota Rav 4, which has been amazing. I tested quite a few cars in the passenger seat and the criteria for me was to be able to turn and swivel into the seat without bending or leaning my body. The Rav is a great workhorse and was a wonderful choice. I am now able to drive short distances and it is perfect.

Not being able to drive was confronting. For me, it represented yet another symbol of my dependency, of isolation and feeling useless. I missed silly things like no longer having the conversations of who was going to have a few drinks that night and who was going to abstain. I was, am, so lucky that I have such a supportive husband who took on the role of permanent chauffeur, amongst his other caring roles, without complaint. Fast forward to 2019, and I started driving again, and with that came a wonderful sense of independence. I still don't drive far, and I always have my phone with me in case I need back up. Driving has without doubt opened up my world again.

And we had to change our bed. That was a big expense. I needed more support and, again, a bed that was high off the ground, so I didn't have far to lower myself, or be lowered. It took a while, as I found going to the shop exhausting and painful, but eventually we found the ideal bed. I'd love to say it has resolved my night pain, but that's not the case. However, having it at the right height makes a big difference to me, especially as I am up many times in the night due to pain and restlessness. We shopped locally, avoiding the gruelling process of parking in a big car park, having to walk on those shopping centre floors and attracting stares from well-meaning shoppers as I hobble like an old woman toward my destination. Apart from the other benefit of keeping local shops in business, the shop owner provided a personalised service, with consideration to my specific requirements.

# Learning about mind, body, soul – and heart

Probably one of the biggest struggles for me to understand was the link between my thoughts, feelings and my pain. As I was navigating my journey, I realised I needed to learn more about the mind/body/soul connection and how by doing this, I could quieten my central nervous system to minimise those pain messages. What I discovered along the way was that I needed to work out what activated my sympathetic nervous system, the flight or fight part of me, and activate my parasympathetic nervous system, the part that helps slow the heart rate, conserve energy and relax the muscles.

This has been the major benefit for me in terms of long-term pain management. You know when we are trying to eat better, to achieve our desired weight and health, the key is to understand the link between mind, body and soul, and to adopt this appreciation and new habits as a lifelong practice, not a six-week 'program'. So often people change their weight by going on a specific, denial kind of diet without understanding the true relationship with their eating patterns. And of course, it's not sustainable. So, hey presto, no surprises that the weight reverts to the 'pre-diet' time, feelings of failure and helplessness abound and one is in a worse position than before the weight change because now there's a whopping pile of guilt and disappointment to add to the low mood and unwanted body shape.

Ditto for pain management. I have found that I have needed to create a new life practice, not an occasional effort. And as I mentioned before, whilst attending the pain programs was beneficial on the one hand, giving me insight into issues such as labelling, language, exercise, etc., having no designated support to continue those practices and increase my understanding of the pain process resulted in the same yoyo affect as what I call 'binge-dieting'.

So, what is the right thing?

There is no right thing – that's my answer. But there is a world of opportunity for each of us to explore how our thoughts, feelings, language and behaviours affect us. That is when you are not brain-fogged with medication, fear or depression. How we clear ourselves of that state is as individual a journey as the uniqueness of our fingerprints. Because our ability to climb out of the mire has to do with four things, in my experience:

- Having the strength and courage to decide that your current state of being is no longer acceptable, and that taking your life is not the get-out clause.
- Having support and love around you – family, friends, health professionals and/or support groups.
- Having the determination to keep learning about your pain and seek answers in places you may never before had thought to look.
- I can find a way to contribute in life, and I acknowledge and respect my determination and resilience.

This is different for everyone. We all have pasts with diverse experiences, and these experiences have moulded our thoughts and behaviours. Some of them are useful, some are not. Some are conscious, most are not. I have created a toolbox of things I can reach into as and when needed: positive self-talk, permission to slow down, and meditation being a few examples. Even saying that I realise I still have a long way to go because many of these strategies in my toolbox need to be everyday occurrences, not just accessed when the flare-ups are threatening or present.

Fundamental to my healing is truly believing that my pain flare-ups were not doing me any more physical damage. That was incredibly difficult, and even now I occasionally doubt it, looking for a mechanical answer to 'fix'. Some habits are really tough to break!

For me, there were two 'aha' moments (well, replace moments with years, but you get the idea) that allowed me to go down this path.

# Using Executive State Identification to Manage my Pain

The first moment sat comfortably with my psychology and behavioural science background, understanding that by shifting my thinking, I could change my thoughts, feelings and to a point, my behaviour. But of course, that is my conscious behaviour I am talking about. Fortunately for me, I have my friend and colleague Jan Sky to thank for this simple yet accurate insight into how I thought about my pain. The following section on Executive State Identification (ESI) provides a snippet of how that played out.

ESI is a mapping tool designed by Jan Sky to map the neural pathways of the brain. The process is goal-directed and allows the client to identify states of behaviour present in given situations. These states have thoughts, feelings and behaviours attached to them and, once identified, self-awareness occurs, and change can happen.

Feeling pain in any part of our body causes distress, and constant chronic pain is debilitating. Managing pain using ESI mapping has been known to relieve pain by shifting the focus from one state to another preferred state. This is best explained by describing how I worked with Jan to map my pain. I knew that whenever the pain struck as a flare-up or a spasm, my thinking would immediately go into 'Fear' mode, anticipating what the next hours, days, weeks or month were going to bring. Fear took over my thoughts, such as, 'Oh shit, here we go again', 'I can't do this anymore' infiltrated my mind.

Jan and I discussed how I could change this, stop the tension, the flight-or-fight reaction that happened each time. By identifying 'Fear' as a state (of mind, of behaviour), Jan asked me if there was another state that had a different profile to Fear that could help manage my pain. It took a while for me to come up with something, feeling that the state of Fear was perfectly reasonable and justifiable. After all, it was evidence-based that a spasm or flare-up ALWAYS resulted in a long stretch of pain, despair, low mood. After some consideration and conversation, I decided on 'Acceptance', recognising that this is what it is and I will get through it somehow, as I always have done. The thoughts I associated with 'Acceptance' were 'I can get through this', 'it's temporary', 'go with the flow', 'breathe and try not to tense my body', 'I do have some level of control over this'.

According to neuropsychotherapy, new neural pathways of the brain are formed at a time when they are most needed in order to support and/or protect us. According to Jan, the state of Fear for me had been formed many years ago when I had my horseriding accident as a teenager; the fear of the pain was real. It has taken me almost 50 years to recognise the fact that by entering the Fear state, I was blocking the opportunity to heal. Accepting that I have some control over the pain was a revelation to me. No point in having a whole lot of techniques up your sleeve if you don't believe they will actually do any good, or if there is a barrier in place, in this case the state of Fear, that inhibits the value of the acceptance.

Of course, like everyone, there are many more states that make up me but acknowledging these two has had a major impact on my pain management. Jan explained that the state of fear stems from the Amygdala, located in the limbic region of the brain, and it would be the 'automatic' response to pain. She calls the Amygdala the 'CEO of negativity', so it makes sense that Fear would seed its beginning here. However, over time, I have developed the state of Acceptance, understanding that this state possibly stems from the prefrontal cortex, the more logical region of the brain. When pain is present and I am aware of Fear, I can choose to focus on Acceptance rather than Fear. This simple process isn't always simple to execute, but when I can, it unequivocally changes the way I think, feel and hence manage my pain.

This self-awareness is a key toward behaviour change. It must be real, authentic and, I have learnt, I must own it; linked with my knowledge that thoughts release chemicals which impact on nerve impulses. I now own my pain, and my ability to manage it to varying degrees, depending on the severity and context of the pain. This is one of many tools in my management portfolio – some days, one or a combination of things works better than others. But we need to have these tools to take back our destiny and our lives.

# Pain and the sympathetic and parasympathetic systems

The second realisation is more complex and an ongoing learning and acceptance. It's about the link between our sympathetic and parasympathetic nervous systems.

Sharon helped me understand the connection between my sympathetic nervous system and parasympathetic system. She added to my understanding of the thinking/nerve-sensitisation connection and suggested ways in which I address these to reduce my sensitised system.

So, what do I mean by a sensitised system?

In brief, and you can read more about this in books I have listed later, the alarm system that feeds the brain pain messages has become so protective that it fires off even when it is no longer actually protecting pain, but results in the same pain message to me. The reason it's often difficult to say exactly where the pain is, (a question so frustratingly, commonly asked by doctors) is because there are no barriers from one nerve connection to another; they are all connected, so the pain spreads across the nervous system, warning me that I am in serious pain. Each movement increases the alarm system's sensitivity, so the more I move, the louder the alarm rings. The problem is, the alarm system is no longer accurate.

Frustratingly, like grief, the pain is often unpredictable and seemingly not related to a particular activity. So, I can appear to be relaxing, or doing what I have always done and not had a problem, and wham, the pain hits me like a brick.

I won't lie, I still get frustrated, but I finally get it. I need to calm my sympathetic nervous system, the one that protects me from threat and pumps adrenalin, and activate my parasympathetic system, the one that helps to slow down my adrenal flow and helps create a state of rest. Because a pain signal happens, my protective mechanism fires up, and that in turns gets all the nerves flying crazily around my body. I visualise this now as a set of old-fashioned scales, constantly seeking balance but always challenged by the loads dumped on each side.

Understanding this is one thing, making it happen is quite another. At this point though, I do want to say that over the years of seeing doctors and pain specialists, maybe one of them mentioned this. I don't know, I can't remember. I do know that it was only when I had the context right that I could hear and understand this message. In other words, for me it was:

- there were no other solutions available
- I was no longer brain mush and so could understand the process

- I had Sharon, a supportive person, to guide me
- I had accepted there was no solution, no cure; it was about self-management.

My biggest active change was the practice of restorative yoga. I tried gentle swimming because I had always loved the feeling of buoyancy in the water and how it cleared my mind. But frustratingly, even the swimming stirs up my system. *Grrr.* And driving there and back was also an activity that could stir me up, so the combination wasn't great. Neil offered to be my chauffeur yet again, but I needed to find something I could do completely for myself.

So, I needed even less energy exertion than gentle swimming or walking in water. Or maybe it was about timing, or building my mind and body in stages – still early days, though I thought there had been many, many long days, months and years. There it is again, that impatience creeping in! I was lucky enough to discover a wonderful yoga teacher at the top of our road. Lise runs a yoga practice, offering a range of yoga styles. Restorative yoga helps the body and mind achieve a state of relaxation and to stop or lessen the constant state of panic and emergency that chronic pain sufferers become wired to experience. This is best explained in the following extract from a Yoga International article:

> Relaxation specifically has been shown to be healing for chronic pain. It turns off the stress response and directs the body's energy to growth, repair, immune function, digestion, and other self-nurturing processes. The relaxation response unravels the mind-body samskaras that contribute to pain and provides the foundation for healing habits. Consistent relaxation practice teaches the mind and body how to rest in a sense of safety rather than chronic emergency.

But it isn't easy. My first few months were really challenging. Getting into the simple lying down positions was difficult and at times caused spasms. I remember a month or so after I started, I was only there ten minutes, my mind was racing, and I became emotional. I tried so hard to be still, but I was flooded with feelings of despair, hopelessness and, even though I was in a room with six others, I felt desperately alone. I couldn't stay lying down as the tears poured down my face. I scrambled up in the most ungainly manner, terrified that my pain was causing a scene, let alone my crazy emotional reaction to, I didn't know exactly what. I left the session, embarrassed as all hell and walked, or rather, hobbled along the streets, hiding behind trees if anyone came my way. I felt terrible. I wasn't going to go home before I was expected because I didn't want to explain to Neil why I was early and so upset. I couldn't explain it to myself. I felt so lost, so overwhelmed with emotion, it was awful.

But I went back the following week, having rationalised my emotions, understanding that by being still, in that moment, I had allowed a pent-up outpouring of loss and grief to overwhelm me. It was real, and to recognise this was a major step toward acceptance and healing. Now, a year later, I can still my mind more often than not and, when I can't, I have learnt to be a witness to it, to not stress about all the brain activity, and just watch it go by. I feel such a sense of achievement in this progress and, without doubt, restorative yoga will be a lifetime practice for me.

And it feels good – no – it feels great, when Lise tells me that I am now an advanced practitioner. Though I don't confuse that with having learnt it all. I hear that as being sufficiently advanced to now achieve a higher level of understanding and practice to continue to activate my parasympathetic system – more simply put, for me to take control (you see, my A-type personality has returned).

On that note, it's not just a once-a-week exercise. Even though classes are weekly, I practice every day, along with meditation and breathing exercises. It's as important to me as the air that I breathe.

I admit to being frustrated when I mentioned to Lise that I would like to join her hatha yoga class she was adamant that I wasn't ready for that.

My first reaction was annoyance; who is she to tell me what I can and can't do? I wanted to do something a bit more active, stretching my body and improving the very limited core strength that I have. But she's right. Because Sharon says the same, and these guys are my barometer when I get a bit carried away.

This week I am sitting in a flare-up. I had to see Sharon again, and she reminded me (as I reminded myself when I screamed and spasmed with the tiniest lean to the left) that I'm in this for the long haul, and gentle-gentle is still my mantra. It's very hard not to push myself when I'm feeling good, but I recognise that it has taken 60 years for my body to reach this state of neural sensitivity – it's going to take the rest of my life to practise desensitising those pathways. And in the main, when I'm feeling positive, I'm OK with that. I accept it.

When I am not in a flare-up, I walk the dogs. I love doing this in the morning. The guys come scrambling out of their 'bedroom', sliding all over the floor as they come to the fridge for their morning treat. They then go out to the garden, have breakfast, and then its walk time. 6.30am. On a good day, Neil walks the big boys and I walk Dougal and Charli. I love these walks and hate to miss them. Mornings are tough because my nights are always disturbed by my pain. Always. Some nights worse than others. Hence, I often feel exhausted in the morning and my body is in pain. However, after I have been up and stretched a bit, walking can be the best remedy: but that's not always the case, and I can never predict how it's going to be. Sometimes it's hard to know if walking will be a good thing or if I am going to get three steps out the front door and be in too much pain to walk. It's the unpredictability that is always a challenge, that I hate, and in a flare-up, the balance between keeping moving, trying to ignore it or stepping back on even the simplest of activities, physical or intellectual, is a constant conundrum.

# Finding My Way Again

As with all journeys, we can look back, reflect and enjoy the beautiful and not so beautiful moments over and over, creating indelible memories in our brains to hopefully share with whoever cares to listen. If we are honest with ourselves, our lives are one long journey, divided into chapters, all of which rely on each other.

At this stage of my journey, I recognise the implicit truth in that process and can identify a few key elements that I know will guide me moving forward.

The first is recognising the importance of acceptance, that what has been is in the past and what is happening now is linked to, but not stuck in those chapters. Accepting the 'Now Dawn' and all that goes with that involves a certain foundation built upon the need to:

- embrace the 'Now Dawn'
- acknowledge that, in accepting this change, there is grief and loss to be acknowledged and worked through

- 'sit with it', to be present in whatever state I was in at the time
- acknowledge that there will be flare-ups
- find joy again
- be a mother, a grandma and a wife again.

Acceptance has been the beginning of my healing. Acceptance is not the same as giving in, it is not giving up. Rather, it's a brave acknowledgement that this is how it is, and to stop fighting. Fighting just activates my neural pathways and makes everything worse. I am proud of my acceptance because it has meant I can seek the support I need to live the beautiful life I have.

Don't get me wrong, Pollyanna is sometimes challenged to the max and I have to fight to keep depression at bay! In many ways, I grieve the 'Then Dawn', but thankfully, not as much as I used to. Here are my key personal learnings from my journey.

# What I had to do to accept the 'Now Dawn'

- Embrace the 'Now Dawn'.
- Acknowledge that, in accepting this change, there is grief and loss to be acknowledged and worked through.
- 'Sit with it', to be present in whatever state I was in at the time.
- Acknowledge that there will be flare-ups.
- Find joy again.
- Be a mother, a grandma and a wife again.

# What I had to grieve before acceptance

- The loss of financial stability that this situation has caused us, and the resultant stress of not knowing how we are going to make it through the next 30 years.
- The spontaneity I used to have, the long walks when my back wasn't playing up and the fact that I could work and play into the wee hours.

- The times when I could be relied on to always 'show up'.
- My career.
- My previous energy levels.
- The ability to plan holidays that are adventures. I am travelling again, but I am wary, I am cautious, and my holidays involve visiting family; I can't do the sightseeing, excursions, etc. I'm not up to that, and because of the unpredictability of my chronic pain, I can't imagine a time when I will be.
- My memory loss – it's frustrating, and I still struggle with short term memory.
- The role of mother and wife as I became the one that my family felt the need to care for, emotionally and physically. And it's hard to get them out of that role, possibly because the pain is still there, and the flare-ups still happen.
- The loss of our sex life – and on the occasion we do get interesting, I pay for it for days or weeks later.
- The loss of my goats – and the opportunity to extend my animal menagerie because it's not fair to

burden Neil with the work if I am unable to look after them.

- I grieve my previous independence, but I am grateful for the level to which it has returned.

## How I have embraced the 'Now Dawn' in ways I could never have imagined

- I have become less judgemental (so much goes on behind my mask that I have no doubt others wear masks to hide their truth).
- I have discovered a peacefulness in myself.
- I am much better at being still, and not feeling guilty about it.
- I am better at self-talk, especially when it comes to keeping depression at bay.
- I appreciate everything around me.
- I am far more connected to my five senses.
- I have learnt so much about chronic pain.
- I feel in control of myself, even when I have the flare-ups.

- I have met some awesome people along this journey.
- I am more creative than I ever was, or perhaps had the time to realise.
- I managed to write and have published my *Oodles of Fun* series of children's books, and have the privilege of them being recognised by the national charity 'Story Dogs' as ideal for children with reading challenges.
- I adore the company of my four dogs – they are the best tonic.
- I have learnt to enjoy my own company.
- I am more realistic about the social occasions I agree to.
- I have learnt, and am excited to keep learning, the benefits of yoga and meditation.
- I can help others along this same journey.
- I have opened my mind to things I never thought were 'me'.
- I have re-established my clinical practice and have started to accept speaking engagements.

# I still find it hard when

- Friends ask me what exactly is wrong with my back.
- I get tired easily.
- I can't do the physical things I loved, and still yearn for.
- Physical touch is so often accompanied with pain.
- Neil can't read my mind!
- The simplest thing like preparing a meal can cause a flare-up.
- I have to wear my mask for an extended period when friends and/or family visit (doesn't mean it's not worth it though).
- I recognise my ability to multitask has been seriously diminished to single, or even half tasks.
- I can't apply for some jobs that look amazing because I will end up over-stimulated and back to square one.
- I must be sensible!

I believe I am well on the way to be the kind of mother, grandma and wife I can be proud of again. I have adopted a new approach, because it is possible since I came off the medication and took back my control. As a mother, I no longer, or rarely, have conversations with my girls about my pain, unless it is obvious by my voice that I am struggling, and they cotton on. Even then, I can honestly say that I am handling it. They don't need to hear that every day I am in pain. They need to know I am OK and that if I needed them, I would say so. They need me to listen to their stories, share their lives, and I am relieved, delighted and so appreciative as I write these words, that is where we are at.

As a grandma, I have adapted what I expect of myself and it's my altered thinking, along of course with my reduced catastrophic, hospital-resulting flare-ups that have revitalised my joy. I don't ask to be with any of the grandchildren on my own, and nor do I allow myself to get into that situation. When the babies are around – how lucky are we, with eight grandchildren to love – I don't even attempt to pick them up. If I want them on my lap or to feed them, I ask for someone to place them on me and to stay close by in case I need to have their beautiful little, but heavy bodies readjusted on my lap, or removed so I can then move. OK, it's not your natural, spontaneous activity and it's frustrating that I can't take responsibility for them so their parents can have a break, but what I have is far better than nothing. And so much better than how it was; so I am grateful.

As a wife, I am much better. I have accepted that there are limits to what I can do, and I am so fortunate to have Neil by my side to not only pick up the slack but ensure there is no slack. I accept that I can give, in so many other ways. I guess what I do find frustrating is when others assume Neil still does everything. That's certainly not the case, not anymore, even though it may not be visible to the outside world!

Emotionally—I have the rest of my life to work on this. I do have my ups and downs but, again, I am much more positive nowadays than a few years ago. I do get anxiety attacks at times but can honestly say that I haven't succumbed to depression in the past few years. I know I am lucky in that way. I do get angry and sad, but I see that as a legitimate reaction to my situation.

Neil is learning to give me space which I appreciate, but the fact that I do not have the energy or nervous system to cope with what I often want to do can create some frustration. I have always been independent, so adapting to his caring and at times overstated concern requires me to take a deep breath sometimes. But hey, what a wonderful challenge to have to face! Reframing what our life is, and can be, is far more of a frustration for me than it is for Neil. His personality is more 'go with the flow' whereas I am, or rather, always was, a 'let's get organised and do it now' sort of person. It's taking time to change, but it's happening.

## Reflections from this Chapter

- Neuropathic pain is nerve damage, often experienced by people with NDRCP.

- We need to learn to manage our pain in a holistic way.
- Taking control of my pain opened up a whole new world of opportunity and discovery – I have hope again.
- I am able to identify what I need and to find joy.
- I take responsibility for the 'Now Dawn'.
- I recognise the impact and connections between my language, thoughts, emotions, physical and social environment.
- I hope I have identified unhelpful habits and created new, helpful ones.
- I am constantly learning about the connection between the sympathetic and parasympathetic nervous system, and what I can do to create balance between them (restorative yoga, regular walking, mindfulness, breathing, meditation, pacing).
- Some things are still hard, but there is a balance to my life now.
- My life is no longer all about my pain.

- I take great pride in sharing my learnings with others through my personal and professional life. My story of despair, loss and resilience now has meaning beyond living with pain.

# Part Four

# Where to From Here?

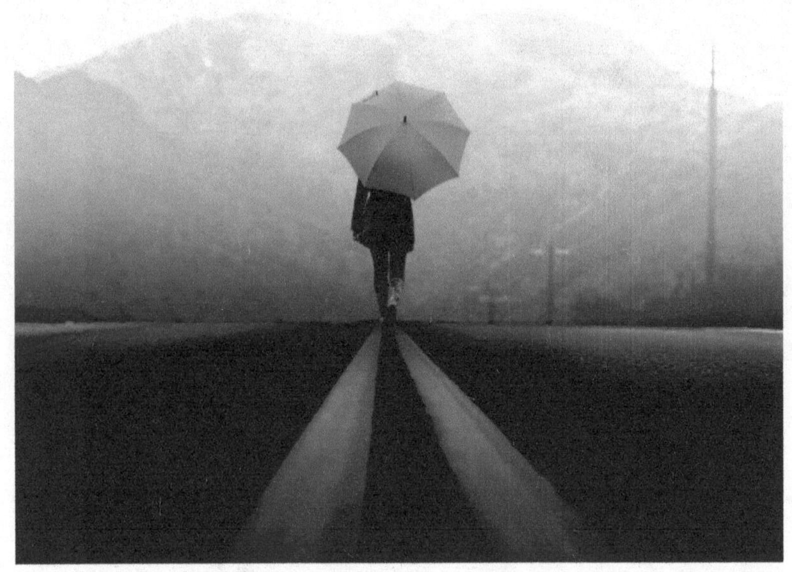

# 10

# FINDING A WAY FORWARD

***Never doubt that a small group of thoughtful, committed, citizens can change the world.***
***Margaret Mead***

In the final section of this book I would like to take the opportunity to say what I think needs to be done to improve the support and reassurance for those of us suffering with nondisease-related, or non-specific chronic pain. I am going to speak out, a bit of the 'world according to Dawn', comforted in the knowledge that in the past few years a lot has changed in the theoretical understanding of chronic pain; specifically, the acknowledgement of the biopsychosocial aspects and the harmful nature of continued opioid use. And whilst there is still a long way to go in health sector practice and community understanding, at least it's being discussed.

In fact, while writing, the Australian government announced that Pain Australia will be supported to develop a National Strategic Action Plan for Pain Management. The Plan will set out key priority areas and measures to improve access to, and knowledge of best practice pain management, in the next three years. This plan includes the importance of community-based support, improved training for medical practitioners and the stigma of chronic pain. More information on the plan is available on the Pain Australia website.

As I mentioned earlier, there are some stark similarities in support needs for those suffering what I referred to in my Doctorate thesis as 'Stigmatised Grief'. So, I will also take the liberty to pop a link to my thesis for anyone that wants to explore that further, as well as list a few books and websites that I have found useful.

# What is Non-Disease-Related Chronic Pain?

Recently, I have heard this referred to as non-specific chronic pain; both terms are useful, and I am encouraged to note that there is finally a label for this condition.

Simply put, pain happens because our brains are responding to what it considers to be a threatening experience. It's all about the message that our nervous system sends to our brain. Sometimes, that message triggers, even when there is no threat evident.

Chronic pain is pain that has continued for three months or more. Often, there is no further actual threat to the body, or any more tissue or skeletal damage, but the pain message still activates in the brain, telling us that the pain is real.

There are many sensory cues that can cause this activation – which is why chronic pain is often frustratingly difficult to describe or predict.

# To all medical and allied health workers

Thank you for everything you do for us. I know you do your best – but none of us know what we don't know. So, this list reflects my experience. Most importantly, I now recognise that even if we ask you and expect you to fix the pain, that's most likely an unfair ask (I am talking about chronic pain here). What we need is for you to also be OK with that, to come to grips with the fact that you can't necessarily fix the pain, but you can help us to manage it. You can reassure us that there is a future for us; we can develop a management plan. *Most importantly, believe us.* Please gently explain in simple language, the slow process toward chronic pain management and support us in a holistic manner. I hope this list is useful and I understand that additional training in chronic pain support, especially the psychosocial aspect of this condition which has such an important influence on our pain, may be required. Sometimes it comes down to something as simple, yet impactful, as the language you use. Remember:

- Our pain is real.
- We are not enjoying this journey.
- Our lives have been totally upended since the onset of this condition.
- How you see us now is not how we were before the chronic pain set in.
- Please validate us and help reduce, not increase, the stigma we feel.
- Please be person-centred – not condition-centred.
- We need to be heard; please take time to listen.
- We probably can't tell you exactly where the pain is because the very nature of non-disease-related chronic pain often results in referred pain, and at times we can't identify 'exactly what we were doing at that time'.
- Our pain experience is different to anyone else's. We are not a 'one size fits all'.
- Please don't think that medications are our only answer.
- Please be very careful with the words you choose. We are a sensitive tribe and any suggestion

that we are making it up, or that the pain isn't as bad as we say it is, just adds to our stress, and therefore, if you understand pain well enough, adds to our pain.

- Maybe you can't fix it. In fact it's more than likely that you alone can't. I know we expect answers, but if you understand pain well you will explain to us gently that chronic pain needs a holistic approach and offer us some supportive pathways.
- Please give us information in a gentle and timely manner. You may have told me things early on, but did I think it was relevant to me? Did I truly understand my chronic pain?
- Please work with us and become one of our team members.
- Please take the time to find other support pathways for us, including modalities such as yoga and meditation.
- Please do not exclude medical cannabis.
- We need ongoing support – counselling by someone who understands non-disease-related

chronic pain, not a generic counsellor or psychologist.

- Support groups can be useful. Do you know of any?
- If you are offering medications, please know that sometimes our side effects are not just those commonly mentioned by the pharmaceutical companies. There are many reasons why one person responds differently to medications than others. Don't dismiss us or say 'just persevere' or put your hands up in resignation.
- Some of the drugs for neuropathic pain are also antidepressants. Please explain to us why you are selecting that specific drug. Otherwise, the message becomes: 'Your pain is not real. You are depressed, it's all in your head'.

A message from my physiotherapist, Sharon—which I believe can be applied to all health professionals:

> Physiotherapists can be challenged by working with people with chronic pain (PWCP). However, when they are able to meet PWCP where they are at, understand them

and get to know them, then everything changes. Once this transformation, which emerges over time, takes place, there is a change from physios feeling as though they are responsible for PWCP getting better and it becomes a facilitating and sharing of the experience of recovery. No one can modulate another's nervous system to desensitise and slow down and be calm all the time. Therefore, physios have had to move away from trying to fix what they have always been taught is a problem in the tissues or structures to move towards helping facilitate long-term relief and improved functioning. This has required a whole change in how physios view themselves and view PWCP in order to provide supportive environments and contexts for living well to minimise ongoing pain.

The change from being an expert in another's body to working in partnership with PWCP and other health professionals who are on the same page is a new way of being for many physios. Some physios struggle with this more than others. Working collaboratively to find what works for each PWCP is empowering and places the PWCP lived experience front and centre in the Physio-PWCP alliance.

I personally feel working with PWCP is an ongoing and emergent process of discovery. The transformational aspects have revealed that with chronic pain there is always more going on than what is seen on the surface. This is in direct contrast to what I was taught a long time ago. I have learnt that working with the uncertainty and novelty of the lived experience of chronic pain requires me to be aware of my own edges of understanding. Therefore I welcome the challenges and feel honoured and privileged to be able to provide whatever support I can as both of us find out how to navigate an intense and often difficult experience.

THANK YOU, SHARON!

# To my friends and family

- Thank you for sticking by me—you know the 'then me' and the 'now me'.
- Please keep asking me to join you doing fun stuff.
- I may not be able to show up every time, but I do want to be included, not cast aside.
- I want to be responsible for making the decision—it's mine to make, not yours (said with love).
- Please be open to a conversation around how you and I communicate about how I am feeling.
- I might need to give you a backup plan in case of a flare-up.
- I don't want your sympathy, but I sure as hell would appreciate your understanding.
- Yes, I welcome suggestions of how other people you know have managed their pain – I appreciate you sharing that with me, but it doesn't mean that if I don't follow that route, I am choosing to not do anything about my pain.

- Yes, I am different now, and in many ways, I embrace the 'now me'. I hope you can too.
- Please don't judge me, I'm hard enough on myself.

## To the community

- Everything I have said above to my friends and family. Especially about the judging.
- Chronic pain is often called 'the invisible disease' so when we park in a disabled car park, please have the decency to accept that we need this space.
- I might look OK to you; in fact, I hope I do. But that doesn't mean I am not struggling or that, due to the unpredictability of my chronic pain, I might flare-up at any moment.
- Please don't gossip about others in pain because we assume you do the same about us!
- If you have a neighbour or member of your community that you know suffers chronic pain, ask them what you can do to help. Then offer

specific suggestions, like a lift somewhere, doing the shopping, cooking or cleaning. Not everyone has the great family support that I have.

## What we need more of

- Counsellors and psychologists trained specifically in the management of non-disease-related chronic pain. We need you to walk alongside us in our journey.
- Physiotherapists and GPs who understand that our pain is unique to us and that we need your guidance to develop a team approach that combines medical and complimentary pathways.
- Physiotherapists and GP's who recognise the importance of a shared management approach to nondisease-related chronic pain; it's not a quick fix, it's a holistic approach to managing our life.
- GP's more open to cannabis prescriptions. It's not fun having to access this as if we are criminals.

- GP's having more time to talk to their patients and get to know them rather than just their presenting pain.
- GP's having access to a database of non-disease-related chronic pain support services that are affordable, or offer Medicare rebates.
- Pathways for ongoing holistic support.
- Non-disease-related chronic pain support groups.
- Greater media awareness of the challenges living with nondisease-related chronic pain; similar to the exposure cancer, heart disease and diabetes are afforded.
- Airtime to keep the challenging issues of living with NDRCP in the public eye, so we de-stigmatise the condition and provide the opportunity for people to have a better understanding, and therefore, offer improved support.
- Increased funding to make all this happen!

In summary – we need to have more open conversations about this condition and see each of us as individuals with a genuine challenge to face. We need a person-centred approach – not to be treated with medications alone because each and every one of us is grieving the loss of life as we knew it and fighting to keep smiling as we recreate ourselves. We can do well, we can acknowledge, embrace and even prefer our 'now' selves. But it's a long road, a road often not of recovery, but more effective management. Our bodies are holding millions of muscle and cellular memories that we need to challenge, and redirect. Thoughts, feelings and emotions are integrated parts of what makes us whole. Reframing all of that takes understanding, acceptance, time and ongoing support.

I am relieved that I am now where I am with my journey, grateful to all those that have walked with me, proud that I didn't give up, excited by what I have learnt and hopeful that my story will help the millions of families in the world that are affected by this life-changing condition.

I sincerely hope that this book has given you and your loved ones essential tools to help you live with your unique and often challenging condition. Know that you are believed. Be strong, be brave and remember the power of one; that even when we feel life is spiralling out of control, there is plenty that we can control, we can influence, and it's up to each and every one of us to help create the change we want to see.

## Reflections

Mirror mirror on the wall
Affixed to one side of the wall
You only see a part of me
One that looks young and carefree

But if you had another side
The one that only the wall could see
Then maybe, just maybe
You'd see the real me

We look in the mirror, we're often so scared
Our body and skin laid open and bare
Is that the person everyone else sees?
Or is that what we show them, just to please

Mirrors reflect life and death
They show a mask, reflect our best
Mirrors only see the light
They don't see what you hide at night

They beam a reflection for all to see
As if all is well between you and me.
But beneath the clear and bright reflection
Lies a person's scared and dark intention.

The life we live is hard to bear
Our daily struggle seems so unfair
It's better to end this agonising life
The pain that cuts through like a knife.

We Photoshop, defy the raw and true
So we don't disturb the love in you
But if you met the real me
You would not like what you could see

You'd probably deny the fact
That it was my true face looking back
You prefer to believe that all is good
And that life is happening as it should

So, I stay behind my mask each day
I don't look in the mirror's way

I work hard to make you smile
And keep you free of all that's vile.

So, when you ask me how I am
You are my mirror; I'll say I'm fine
And you can go about your life
Without the burden of my strife.

I hope one day I'll have a mirror
That smiles back at me with love and fervour
But until that time, the show must go on:
Yes, life is good, there's nothing wrong.

# ACKNOWLEDGEMENTS

This book has been an epic journey for me, one that I couldn't possibly have survived without some amazing people in my life.

To Big Sky Publishing, for believing in me and recognising that my story is one that speaks for millions and needs to be told. And thank you for putting me in touch with Sean. Sean through your professionalism, firm, scary and awesome editing advice, you have made my story into everyone's story. Thank you.

To Kay, we have travelled so many roads together. Through trauma, professional support, awesome writing insights and friendship, we are there for each other when it matters. Ours is something pretty unique. Thank you.

To my friends who have stuck with me along my life journey, I hope my words in this book show you just how important your continued love and support have meant to me.

A heartfelt message of love and thanks to my family. All of you have watched me through the light and the dark times. You have felt helpless as you shared my pain, which I know became your pain. We have become stronger through it all and I love you forever.

Lorraine, thank you for being bold enough to help me focus on the important aspects of my story, so my story can belong to everyone. It was a tough process, but absolutely worth it. Thank you.

And to Neil. You appeared in my life when times were tough. It got tougher, for both of us and we have come out smiling and stronger than we ever thought was possible. You are my best friend, my soul mate and my rock. I love you.

# Appendices

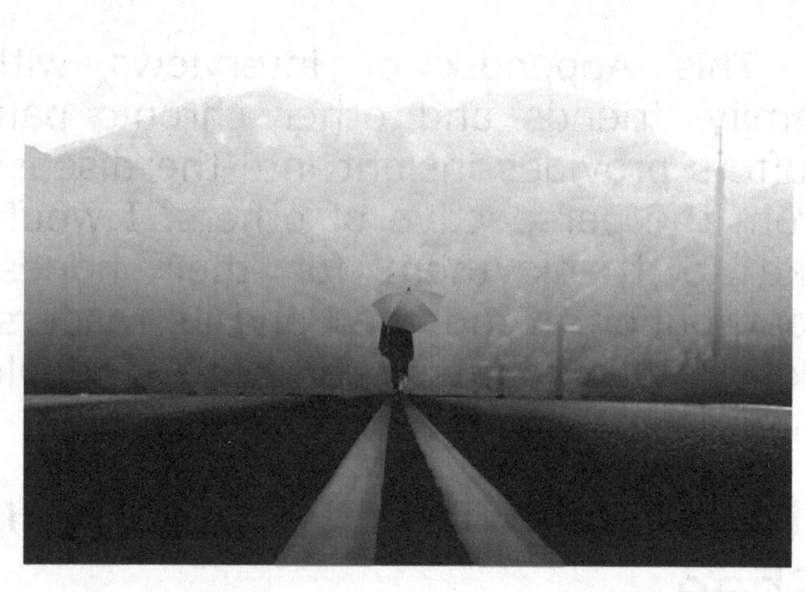

# APPENDIX 1

# BEHIND THE MASK: CONVERSATIONS AND INTERVIEWS

This Appendix of interviews with family, friends and other chronic pain suffers provides insight into the disease from the perspective of others. I would like to thank them for their honest contribution to the book and its readers. Note the names of the people interviewed have been changed.

## Interview with my daughter, Shae

**How, if at all, does my pain affect you?**

On your worst days, you shut yourself away. You stay in your room, shut the door, both literally and emotionally.

I know, even if it's over the phone, that you are not good. But what's worse for me is when I see you in pain.

I remember coming home from our honeymoon. There was this old woman barely shuffling toward us, like a 90-year-old, bent over with effort. Everyone was looking.

I sat there with Jon and wanted to cry. It was so difficult. We had just returned from our honeymoon, in our wedded bliss, wanting to share the photos with you guys. Seeing you dripping in sweat because the pain was so intense. Seeing you gritting your teeth, trying to get through the moment – who were you trying to convince, you or me?

Seeing you in so much pain was gut-wrenching. Neil had driven you from Byron Bay. You made it to the table we were sitting at but could barely get yourself into the seat. Neil went to buy a cushion from the shop down the road to help you get a bit more comfort; I ran in front of him, needing to compose myself, as well as explain to the shopkeeper that we only needed to borrow the cushion – not buy it. I remember she kindly lent it to us, having seen you cross the road. Neil lovingly placed the pillow behind your back.

When it's meant to be a good day, and it turns into a bad day – that's the hardest to see.

I see a snippet of the really bad, and then you lock yourself away. It's your protection mechanism for us. You don't want us to see you in so much pain. So, we don't ever see the whole pain, the extreme pain. You lock yourself away from those you love so we don't see the pain – trying to protect us.

That's why when we are out together, walking around the shops or markets, and then the pain hits you – you are stuck. You can't lock yourself away. That's the hardest.

I can't ever forget the image of you shuffling across the road, all the cars stopped, eyes watching you, not with a 'get off the road' look, but a 'why isn't this young woman in a wheelchair – she's obviously in so much pain?' look. But how do I help? None of us knows where to start.

You sit there and look on. It's like your feet, your whole body is locked in concrete. You know you can't help. No Panadol is going to make it go away. You can't help.

It's the worst, most useless, gut-wrenching feeling I've ever had.

# Susan, 42 years old, Endometriosis, Adenomyosis, Motor Vehicle Accident

I have two sources of chronic pain. I have lived with the first, endometriosis and adenomyosis, from the onset of menstruation. In 2009 I had a motor vehicle accident which left me with multiple fractures, internal injuries and minor petrol burns.

I am in chronic constant pain, every day. From the moment I wake up the first thing my brain/body is aware of is that I am in pain. Throughout the day I can be struggling to find physical positions to be able to work at a computer to perform my job.

I have difficulty at times focusing due to the pain, particularly with break-through-pain or a pain flair and I get severe migraines.

Despite the bone crushing exhaustion and fatigue, the pain still keeps me awake at night.

As with other types of pain, endometriosis and adenomyosis pain flares occur without logical reasoning; at times when I am severely unwell, I collapse. I am acutely aware of almost each and every cell in my body. I can feel the endometriosis growing and changing inside. I know when my body reaches this point, my whole self (all systems) cannot continue and I need surgery again.

When experiencing a pain flare, I am mostly bedbound, and it renders me unable to function either at work or to complete day-to-day tasks. I developed an opioid intolerance after surgery in 2017, which makes daily pain management even more challenging.

There is pain sitting, moving and when lying down, pain with bladder function, when opening the bowels, or pain passing wind, (which is common with endometriosis and adenomyosis), generalised pelvic pain, excruciating back pain (like being chopped with an axe), painful bloating, pain when ovulating, painful (excruciating) periods, excessive bleeding, pain during or after sex, painful clotting, painful pelvic spasm, barbed-wire pain through the legs (some gynecologist believe it is only felt with women who have small or large intestine endo legions, others don't know).

Non-pain related symptoms (that cause mental, emotional and daily life related pain) are brain fog, infertility, vomiting, night sometimes day sweats, having trouble holding a full bladder or frequently emptying the bladder (I have both endo on the bladder and adhesions which super-glued the bladder and uterus), restless leg syndrome at night when trying to sleep, severe headache and or migraine, sleeplessness, etc.

For some people with endometriosis, the pain is minor and doesn't intrude too much on their lives. For others, like me, the pain flares up regularly and can be really debilitating.

I have had multiple surgeries; the first when I was 23 and most recently at 40. I also take a range of medications to manage the pain.

The only permanent option for adenomyosis is a full hysterectomy which I won't consent to at the moment. I have tried zoladex for the past seven months, which has actually significantly assisted in pain management however, the side effects were quite horrific, even brutal, and I needed HRT to help. This treatment has been ceased, and I have started Endep – a first generation anti-depressant that can assist some women with chronic pelvic pain.

In addition to the above I eat a dairy free, plant-based diet, supplemented by vitamins.

My pain is exacerbated by the multiple fractures that occurred as a result of my accident. I have osteoarthritis in my back, my body is stiff, and I have difficulty at times walking despite osteo treatments and cortisone injections.

My experience has been outstanding with professors and surgeons who are also actively engaged in the academic chronic pain management field. GPs generally don't understand these diseases, and therefore their capacity to help manage pain can be very limited. I have been asked numerous times by GPs if I am a doctor (no, I'm just informed about what these diseases are doing to my body, and what the results of the motor vehicle accident have done). My current GP is the best one I have even had and is pivotal to the on-going management of my health.

I also have a psychologist who I have been seeing for the past five and a half years which is absolutely critical in my ability to manage my life and body/pain.

On a good day, I get out of bed without too much pain, and it helps if I have slept the night before. I achieve what I need to without being clouded in pain fog. I can eat, I may even laugh or feel 'OK'.

A bad day starts with a headache when I open my eyes, they burn, and I feel nauseous. I may vomit, I may walk into the wall trying to use the bathroom, my mouth is dry, and I feel awful. I am hollow, like I am somehow detached from my body.

I try to do what I need to; sometimes I have trouble with my legs and cannot feel them very well. I will not be able to think clearly or concentrate on days like this, but I will go to work, and do the study that I need to do in order to keep functioning.

I can't take painkillers more than paracetamol/ibuprofen so I will do that, to take the sharp edge off. I would like to stay in bed with a hot water bottle, but I need to work, and I have study commitments. My brain is sometimes appreciative of the distraction from my physical pain that doesn't stop.

I try to block the pain out and stay focused on what I have to achieve for the day. A glass of wine at lunch sometimes helps, I stretch in my office. I try to accept the pain instead of trying to get rid of it. I learned many years ago that I had to surrender.

My chronic pain has affected my life in many ways. It has been detrimental to my work and career and relationships are compromised. I don't often socialise as I am struggling to maintain energy for my daily life let alone get into conversations with people that I don't know. As my diseases are invisible, it's hard to explain why I am so exhausted and that I may 'want' to participate but can't imagine how.

After being single for the past five years, I have a new partner. I know he hopes things will work out, and I feel better but beyond that I am unsure how the future will unfold.

There are some positives from my situation. I am much stronger and more resilient and feel like I know myself inside and out. I have complete awareness of my body being 'ok, well, average, poorly, excellent' due to a baseline of standard capacity that I doubt I would have attained otherwise.

I can understand complex medical issues and I have refused to give in to my disabilities, or inabilities.

A major benefit is that I have learned how to identify gratitude: in others, circumstances, and in myself. I recognise the need to surrender to the pain, give the pathways colours even, accept it, don't try to get rid of it. The more you fight, the bigger it gets.

I know that I have a responsibility to be the best version of myself that I can be.

## Paul, Spinal Injury

In 1998 I was a relief Captain on a Boeing 747-400 aircraft when I injured my spine due to an in-flight assault by a passenger. The injury was then exacerbated years later as a result of repetitive sitting and twisting in the cockpit seat. My subsequent back surgery failed, leaving me with chronic pain and PTSD.

I have a constant thumping, burning and tingling pain in my lower back which varies in intensity. My pain score can be between 2 and 8 depending on the day. But a lot of the time, it's a 10 on the pain score. I have psychogenic blackouts and pain attacks which feel like a lightning bolt starting in the lower back and then shooting up my spine and down to my right leg. These are so intense I normally black out with the pain, resulting in more injuries. When I come to, I often have damage to my head. Because of these psychogenic blackouts, over the years, I have required countless stitches to my head and face and received multiple surgeries. I have damaged both knees and have needed a meniscus repair operation. I have also broken my right hand, right wrist and left cheek.

My chronic pain is relentless. I feel it twenty-four hours a day seven days a week. It wakes me in the night. I have no relief from it. It just takes over completely, destroying you bit by bit.

It consumes me to the point I have little capacity to think about or do anything else. I was once a completely independent man and now I need assistance in dressing, showering, toileting and taking my many medications. Things that I used to enjoy like housework, cooking, gardening and other normal day to day activities are no longer achievable. I lost the ability to have any sex life after my lumbar vertebral body replacement surgery in 2013. I live in a constant state of anxiety, fearful of the next fall or inevitable pain attack – knowing it is only a matter of time before experiencing yet again, the excruciating painful episodes that comes with chronic pain. I experience terrifying PTSD flashbacks which add to my anxiety. It's a terrifying experience to come out of a flashback and finding yourself back in reality. I fight with my depression every day and the suicidal thoughts of just wanting the pain to stop. Forever.

I am completely dependent on my wonderful wife who is now my full-time carer and get frightened and fret when I am not with her. If she can't be with me one of my children takes over the role for a short time. Before everything, my friends would describe me as energetic and happy but now I am in such a dark and frightening place, I just want the pain to stop. You become so consumed, worn out and empty that you don't think rationally or about the consequences. And so I have attempted multiple times to end my suffering. The guilt that comes after these attempts is overwhelming, but at the time you don't think about that. You don't think about how ending your own suffering would cause more suffering for your family. My family knows this and they are the reason I am alive today.

I am so lucky to have such an incredible wife and three supportive children, as well as some great friends and a team of doctors all dedicated to helping me.

Every day I yearn for a normal life and hope one day that there will be a cure for me but I still struggle trying to be positive and to be grateful for what I have.

I have had numerous surgical interventions as well as medication for pain and PTSD.

I seem to have a 3-month cycle at the moment where the pain medications stop working and the pain becomes so unbearable, then the only option left is hospitalisation for intervention.

I have mixed experience of the medical profession. I have met some really wonderful dedicated doctors, and then there are the rest. I am so lucky to have such a tremendous team of doctors treating me now, who are at the top of their field and are extremely knowledgeable and compassionate, caring and always go that extra mile for me. However, my past experiences have left me feeling despondent and in despair. I feel like I have been failed by the profession and that previous doctors didn't uphold their ethical oath of doing no harm. I feel like they broke me and put me back on the shelf and didn't care to try and fix me.

I have had brilliant counselling and psychiatric support. They have given me strategies to help me cope with my 'new reality'. I have been taught to use a therapy called 'mindfulness'. This is a fantastic tool to use with dealing and helping to cope with chronic pain on a daily basis.

I have very few good days however when I do have them it looks like this:

My wife wakes me up and administers my morning medications with a glass of milk to avoid nausea. I then might doze for another 30 minutes to an hour, building up the strength to get out of bed. She will then help me go to the toilet.

I try and help with breakfast by chopping something sitting down but I usually just watch her and talk about our plan for the day. She will then shower and dress me. We will then put on some relaxing music and try and do some mindfulness or meditation. On a really good day, my wife will walk our dogs while I ride beside her on my electric scooter. If we can't do that, I'll try and throw the tennis ball a few feet for my dogs to play catch with. I can't do much for them, but they do SO much for me.

We have lunch and my medication. We have to stick to a rigid drug schedule otherwise the pain becomes unbearable. We try and invite friends over for coffee or lunch but it's difficult as it's a touch and go situation. We might make plans in the morning and have to cancel them later on which has left social situations a rarity. Only real friends understand our situation and sadly we have lost many 'friends' as they grow tiresome of our sporadic plans.

Then we go to hydrotherapy or something else to get us both out of the house. We might even try and meet our kids out for lunch if I can manage it.

I spend the late afternoon recovering by lying on the couch and watching a bit of TV, usually with my dogs by my side or even on the couch with me!

After dinner we'll put a nice movie on to finish off our day. It doesn't sound like much but just being together means everything to me. My wife will then help me change and get into bed and gives me my night-time medication.

My bad days are really bad days. I can't even get out of bed and require so much more medication, both for pain and mental health, that I have accidently overdosed a few times. I try and sleep these days away, but I wake up in hot and cold sweats, become incontinent and become a shell of the person I am. Sometimes these days are strung together, and a week can go by. I'm just very grateful I have my family who pull me out of these days.

My pain has affected my life in every way. I was a senior international airline Captain with over 33 years of flying experience and was medically retired/terminated basically overnight. I still had over 12 years left, before reaching the legal age of retirement, to continue my successful career. To have my profession, independence and health taken away from me, through no fault of my own, was heartbreaking.

My family and I were not financially ready for me to retire and due to the ongoing medical and legal bills, we have lost everything we own. Our home, superannuation, savings and shares. Our out-of-pocket expenses keep going out with no income coming in. This adds an overwhelming amount of stress onto us that we really can't cope with.

Due to my pain and mental health, I am now very reluctant to leave the house. I used to love socialising and events but now I can't even go to a football game without crippling anxiety attacks. We mostly stay at home to both save money and our emotions.

I struggle with my sense of self-worth. I used to be the confident, and independent bread winner and now my wife has to do everything for me. My career was a big part of my identity and now that I don't have that, I struggle with self-love and purpose. It's really tough.

My pain has affected my wife in every way. She has had the hardest job adapting to our new life. She has had to give up her career in order to become my full-time carer. Her whole life has been turned upside down. She has to balance being a mother, wife, friend and now carer as well. Due to my disabilities, Ruth has had to attend every doctor appointment, physio session and hospital stay, just to name a few. She has not only lost her own personal time and independence, she doesn't have the opportunity for separation from me. She also has no escape from our life, whereas I can take medications when things get too much, stay in bed or go to hospital.

My situation has also greatly affected her own health. She spends all her time so worried about me that she forgets to look after herself and consequently her health has suffered. She suffered a stroke brought on by stress in 2018 and I feel responsible.

I am so lucky to have such a loving strong supporting woman in my life. We met as teenagers and have been together ever since. It takes a very special person to stick around. A lot of couples split when you consider all the stresses, both financial and emotionally, the frustration, the sadness and the disappointments we have had to endure, over these very long last eight years.

My view on life, although cynical, due to my condition, has changed for the better. I remember the sayings, 'your health is your wealth' or that 'your health is the most important thing in life' but I took those for granted and didn't act accordingly. Now, I have taken a step back and had a long hard look at what really matters in life. It isn't money or power, it's health and love and our family and friends that are essential for a full and happy life. I am so lucky to still have all these things.

Due to my flying career, I missed out on so many important events and milestones. It has been a blessing to be able to now be there for birthdays, Christmases, and other important family events. This is something that for 35 years, wasn't guaranteed.

The hardest changes have been to try and accept my new reality (still a work in progress). For me, this is loss of identity, energy, concentration, control, independence, dignity, financial security. I also struggle to accept that I am in this position through no fault of my own.

I have attended many pain clinics in Brisbane and Melbourne and as such met with many people dealing with chronic pain. Sadly, several of them have lost their fight and taken their own lives. Sadly, too many people haven't had the support I've had, and as a result have lost their brave fight. The average person does not comprehend what pain does to people. Like with mental health, there is no bandage to show. Chronic pain is an invisible disease and it lacks empathy from healthy people. The stress, the disappointments, the inability to cope with everyday life, is such a struggle. Whilst you need help from the medical fraternity and daily medication, the most important thing to have is the loving support of your immediate family. That is what keeps you alive – to be with them, for them.

# Rachel, Paul's wife and carer

When Paul had his spinal surgery back in 2011, I wasn't prepared for any other outcome other than a full recovery. However, that wasn't the case for us. Following many failed surgeries, Paul spent an enormous amount of time in hospital. If memory serves, it must have been over 11 weeks in a row at one point. I visited him every day. Sometimes he wouldn't wake and sometimes he would forget I was ever there due to the amount of drugs they had him on. But I did it so I could encourage him to eat if he could. His body was frail, and as the weeks went on my once solid husband had lost over 45 kilos and looked like a bag of bones. I was lost for words at the unhelpful staff, who didn't see it as their job to ensure the patient ate. So, every day I would encourage him to eat.

Paul was eventually relocated to a hospital closer to home, the family was delighted and it seemed he was on the road to recovery at last. Two weeks later he was discharged to our home. He was told to have regular blood tests to watch out for the Golden Staph infection returning. Little did we know that his levels were already at a dangerous and unacceptable reading. Within two weeks Paul's CRP levels were so dangerous that our eldest son had to rush him back to the main hospital in Brisbane for immediate attention. Where was I during this? At the vet with our other son and daughter euthanizing our precious but very sick golden retriever. This was just the beginning of the compromises our family have had to make to ensure Paul's wellbeing.

After roughly 18 months of what seemed like a spinning wheel of doctor appointments and disappointments, Paul's company terminated his employment and deemed it 'medical retirement'. Paul's successful career was always so heavily intertwined with his identity. So for Paul, losing his career was like losing a part of him. He was emotionally grieving and also battling physical pain. Overnight, I became a counsellor with no warning and with no prior training.

It has now been seven years since the Golden Staph infection invaded his spine and our entire world has changed. I have had to learn a lot of medical terms, resorting to books and the internet when I didn't understand a diagnosis. I hide away some of the drugs as Paul had overdosed previously and dispensed them himself when he can't cope with the pain. I have put him to bed every night, heated up heat packs for him when he needs them and even participated in a mindfulness course with him. Anything to help him.

I drive Paul to his various appointments and need to sit with him as he has memory losses and trouble understanding what is going on. I have had to endure every painful step as he retold his story to psychiatrists, psychologists, doctors and nurses over and over again. I held his hand every step of the way and have spoken for him when he lost his train of thought, often, due to the cocktail of opiate medications he is on. Twenty-four hours a day I basically have to do everything for Paul. I do this without hesitation however, sometimes it gets very hard when I'm ill, and still having to cope helping Paul as well. It does get overwhelming at times, but I am so very lucky to have a supporting daughter and sons to take over when I need assistance. Most people don't really understand that Paul's chronic pain is relentless day in and day out, and the struggle I have with trying to keep him, as well as myself, positive.

Our family was not financially ready either of us to retire and due to the ongoing medical and legal bills, we have lost everything we own. Our home, superannuation, savings and shares. Our out-of-pocket expenses keep going out with no income coming in.

Although, I do not blame Paul for us being in this situation, he still feels that he has let the family down. On some occasions Paul has expressed his desire to end his pain and suffering forever and has acted on these feelings. It is beyond difficult to hear these things coming from a loved one and even harder to pick up the pieces. I try to calm Paul through positive distraction. We grow herbs and small vegetables and cook lots of lovely meals and have even mastered pickled onions in an attempt to keep busy. I have to remind Paul on a daily basis that it is not his fault and that together we can get through anything. But sometimes I have doubts about the future, and that makes me sad as well. It's hard lifting someone else up all the time when you yourself feel so down.

Living with someone in chronic pain has affected my life in so many ways, but the biggest impact would be that of my own health. I worry for Paul's so much that I neglect my own. The constant stress and uncertainty of our situation resulted in my own health struggles and in February 2018 I suffered a stroke. I had a pacemaker inserted shortly after and am doing okay but it has knocked me. I do what I can to move forward and try to wake up every day and write down five things I am grateful for.

A little while ago I came across the following song. It's an old one by the Pretenders but I think it sums up my life with Paul now. The first verse resonates deeply with me.

*Oh, why you look so sad, the tears are in your eyes,*
*Come on and come to me now,*
*and don't be ashamed to cry,*
*Let me see you through,*
*because I've seen the dark side too,*
*When the night falls on you, you don't know what to do,*
*Nothing you confess could make me love you less,*
*I'll stand by you.*
*I'll stand by you, won't let nobody hurt you,*
*I'll stand by you.*

## Hannah, 64 years old, Shoulder Injury

My pain started five years ago, a few months after a shoulder injury. I had a torn rotator cuff, frozen shoulder and calcium spur. I became intolerant to all medications, so I had to reduce all my meds which increased my stress. I also have developed complex regional pain syndrome (CRPS) – which has all led to Fibromyalgia.

It's affected me in many ways; I'm reluctant to make plans to go out because I don't like to cancel and let people down. If I do go out, I often don't enjoy it because of the pain and tiredness I feel. It affects my marriage and all other relationships.

I've tried numerous pain management strategies, acupuncture, alternative doctors, neurologists, counselling, Emergency Departments, physiotherapists and rehabilitation programs. Counselling has been the most helpful, supported by mindfulness techniques. I also have massages when I can tolerate them and my husband and I go to Gestalt therapy together. I also do trauma release exercises and I practice meditation, reminding myself that this won't last. I try to be more centred and not catastrophise.

The balance between good and bad days varies. I can have a few good days, even weeks and months. Then if my stress increases, my inflammation increases too, and it all starts up again.

On a good day I have reasonable energy with little or no pain. My anxiety is low and so I feel I've got myself back again. Consequently, I feel happy.

But on a bad day I feel black emotionally, despondent and in a lot of pain. I get little sleep, feel nauseous, and have limited mobility.

My sense of worth has been affected. I feel shame and guilt because I feel like I am a burden. Before, I was always confident and able to contribute financially. Now I feel deep sadness. I have pulled away from friends. I don't have much to talk about-I feel detached, isolated. It's very distressing for my husband, he can't fix it. He feels like he has lost the joyous part of me; we don't have a lot to say to each other anymore.

I have become more of a negative person, which I don't like. Not all the time, but it's easy to get into that place. I can't do long travel trips. Last time we did, it was too difficult. It pulls me back into a bad place, physically and mentally.

There have been positive outcomes. I have more empathy for people struggling with mental illness as I am now experiencing emotional pain. I read a lot and try to educate myself. I have to adjust goals around the immediate and be OK with that. I have improved my self-care, which is positive. I'm not sure about the future – at the same time, I try not to ponder.

## Mandy, 60 years old, Spinal Fracture

When I was 12 years old, I had a severe skiing accident resulting in open spiral fracture in my leg. I had a 9-kilo cast for two and a half months which unsettled my pelvis. Sciatica set in at 15 years old and

I then had chronic fatigue in my late 20's, though in those days, it wasn't recognised. It took three to four years to improve. I did a lot of alternative treatment.

The sciatica then became a big issue in my second pregnancy, 23 years ago. I had shoulder pain, sciatica, hip pain and double scoliosis. It was like a severe, sharp knife pain. My pelvis and tailbone were so painful, I couldn't sit for three months after the birth. My coccyx was really bent.

By the time I was 40, I had so much pain in my body. When I was 18 in Africa, I lost 15 kilos – I had dysentery and Giardia. It was like an onslaught and has affected my pain because I can't absorb foods in the optimum way. So, in addition to sciatica, I now have osteoporosis and a compromised system.

It's been devastating not to be seen, heard, met or believed. I have been fearful and anxious that I have had something terrible that the doctors have missed.

I shared these feelings with my partner, but he could only sympathise.

I have found a serious lack of expertise. I have had some surgery, but I see it as a last resort. The medical model of medication has too many side effects, so I stay clear as much as possible.

I have learnt many alternate treatments myself. It comes in many forms; my food, vitamin and mineral supplements and B12 injections for energy. I don't eat sugar.

I use liquid herbs from the naturopath to settle the gut. Blastocysts. I have pain from the osteoporosis which affects my sleep. There is a definite connection between gut health and pain.

I also see an osteopath, chiropractor and massage therapist.

I haven't sought counselling support for physical pain, but I have looked in books, and online.

On a good day I manage four to six hours of clinical work. My work has been on and off – so I definitely have a reduced income. I have less capacity to work but have adjusted to that. Morning pain is par for the course. I believe my aqua aerobics is a big help and I realise the energy I have to cope with the pain. I consciously admit the pain to myself, but don't mention it to others.

A bad day is DISAPPOINTING! When I have physical pain it affects my mind. If I can't be sharp and clear, I get frustrated and devastated that this day is like this.

I manage a bad day by accepting it and employing distraction techniques. I have managed before; I can do it again. Self-talk. Having something to look forward to later; a book perhaps or a film. Looking forward gives me joy – it takes away the emotional greyness of that day.

I am very discerning who I talk to about my troubles. There are some people that I never talk to about my pain. My partner has never known me without pain. I'm good at dealing with it, at hiding it although I am often exhausted.

Between 40 and 50 I wasn't as capable as I should have been; my sense of self was hugely affected. Lots of judgement, 'should, should, should'. I put pressure on myself which resulted in increased pain and I got into a very bad cycle. Living with chronic pain is fatiguing on a daily basis. I used to lie about my situation so others didn't judge me. I realise this was an internalised stigma because I was embarrassed to admit I didn't do much.

My condition has affected my view of the future. I recognise that my home is my safety net and have less curiosity about the outside world . If I travel, I get worried, fearful – 'what if?' It's scary, lonely.

I find myself underplaying and undermining myself. It's very hard to explain to someone who doesn't understand. I start to feel the 'wobbliness' of our culture – it has to have a name, a diagnosis for that to be true!

I don't talk to friends about it; I feel like it's too hard to explain, 'Here I am again'.

I do find as my friends get older and are experiencing ageing pain, they understand more – but not 20 years ago.

# APPENDIX 2

# MY PAIN CYCLE – PROBABLY THE SAME AS MOST PEOPLE'S!

## My Pain Cycle

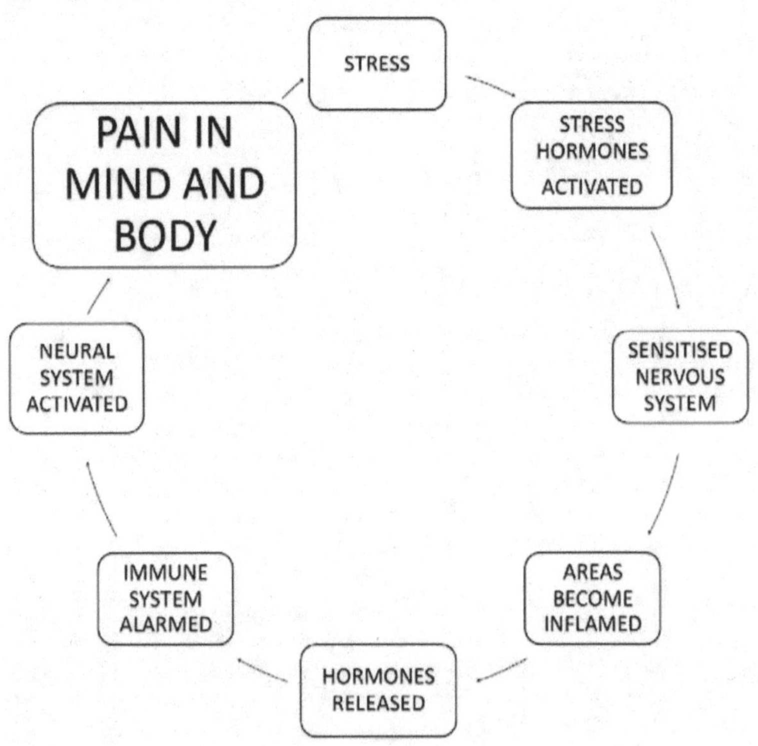

# Pain out of control

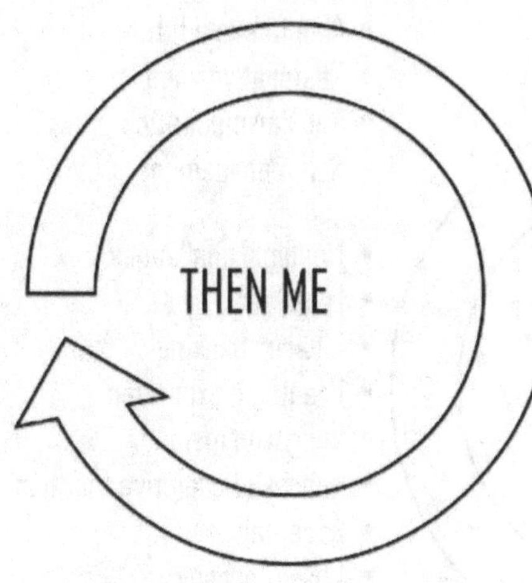


- Opioid dependent
- Constant GP visits
- Isolation
- Suicidal ideation
- Depression
- Multiple specialists
- Acupuncture
- Physiotherapy
- Xrays, CT scans
- Medically induced stroke
- Memory loss
- Impaired cognitive function
- Exhaustion
- Brain fog
- Fear
- Financial crisis
- Rehabilitation
- Repeated ED visits
- In-hospital admissions

# Pain in control

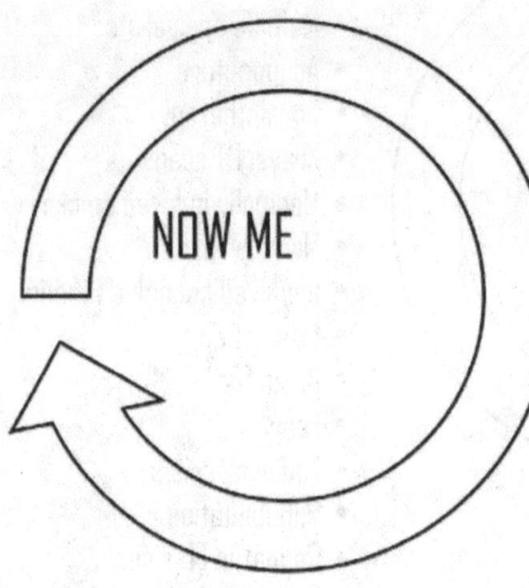


- Occasional GP visits
- Improved social life
- Improved mood
- Able to see a future
- Restorative yoga
- Regular meditation
- Self management of flare ups
- Finanical challenges
- Less fear
- Clearer thinking
- Breathing exercises
- Improved memory
- Improved cognitive function
- Acceptance
- Physiotherapy
- Improved communication
- No more opioids
- Pacing and being realistic
- Adapting
- Plant based diet to reduce inflammation
- Reflexology

# APPENDIX 3

# THREE USEFUL THERAPIES FOR PAIN MANAGEMENT

## 1. Eye Movement Desensitisation and Reprocessing, (EMDR)

Eye Movement Desensitisation and Reprocessing, EMDR for short, is a therapy established for people – children as well as adults who have had traumatic experiences. It is also helpful for a variety of emotional, physical and behaviour problems in adults and children. There is a wealth of information about current research available on the EMDR Association of Australia website.

EMDR is a World Health Organisation recommended treatment for Post-Traumatic Stress Disorder (PTSD).

EMDR is an approach that seems to help 'unblock' the brain's processing so that traumatic memories can become 'ordinary' memories. We do not know precisely how this treatment works. It may have something to do with the alternating left-right stimulation of the brain – or with REM sleep in which the eyes often move from side to side on their own.

Research now shows that physical pain can be linked to either unresolved PTSD from trauma or has in itself become a traumatic experience. Understanding how to work with the underlying trauma, as well as the subjective experience of pain frames the way EMDR approaches this subject.

EMDR therapy is protocol-based therapy i.e. it has rules! Therefore, when working with those experiencing pain the therapist will employ both the standard protocol for trauma, and also a specific pain protocol.

The EMDR therapist will help a client to process the underlying neurological responses which contribute to the pain, develop strong strategies for coping with on-going pain, and process any traumatic experiences which are feeding the pain response in the body.

In summary, research indicates that EMDR can facilitate pain relief and reduce the emotional distress associated with the trauma associated with pain.

**Jackie Gess EMDR Accredited Practitioner, MBACP Accredited Counsellor**

## 2. Acceptance and Commitment Therapy

People with chronic pain often avoid situations or activities that they expect to cause or increase their pain, as well as the distressing thoughts and emotions about themselves and their lives that can become as difficult to live with as the chronic pain. Such avoidance often leads to a life that gets narrower and narrower, until it has little in common with the person's former life. Acceptance and Commitment Therapy, or ACT (pronounced like the word 'act'), helps people to move purposefully towards their valued goals even though they live with chronic pain.

According to ACT, it makes sense to try to cope with chronic pain using avoidance and control, because avoidance is a natural consequence of our ability to evaluate, predict and avoid events. The problem is that avoidance and control are ineffective strategies for managing internal experiences like troubling thoughts, emotions or chronic pain.

The ACT therapist and client uncover all of the strategies the client has used to manage their pain, and the client considers whether those strategies have moved them closer to or further away from the things that matter to them. This exploration leads the client to recognise that avoidance and control haven't worked. This opens the door for the therapist to propose a different approach to living with chronic pain: accepting the experience one is having, however unpleasant, and as much as possible in a given situation, acting in ways that take them closer to the things they value.

To facilitate this, the ACT therapist teaches the client six core skills: Acceptance of internal experiences (instead of avoiding them); cognitive diffusion (changing the relationship to thoughts and feelings); defining valued directions (which can guide one's actions), being present (instead of living in the past or in an imagined future), committed action (choosing and taking actions that align with values), and self as context (seeing the self as an observer of experience, rather than self as the experience itself). The aim of all of the skills is to increase the individual's psychological flexibility – their ability to persist with behaviours that align with their values, without avoiding or trying to control unpleasant experiences. **Cecelia Titus, MSc, BSc.**

## 3. Cognitive Behavioural Therapy (CBT)

Cognitive behavioural therapy (CBT) is a form of talk therapy that helps people identify and develop skills to change negative thoughts and behaviours. CBT says that individuals – not outside situations and events – create their own experiences, pain included. And by changing their negative thoughts and behaviours, people can change their awareness of pain and develop better coping skills, even if the actual level of pain stays the same.

What can CBT do for you? Cognitive behavioural therapy helps provide pain relief in a few ways. First, it changes the way people view their pain. Joseph Hullet MD, a leading medical expert on CBT says, 'CBT can change the thoughts, emotions, and behaviours related to pain, improve coping strategies, and put the discomfort in a better context'. You recognise that the pain interferes less with your quality of life, and therefore you can function better.

CBT can also change the physical response in the brain that makes pain worse. Pain causes stress, and stress affects pain control chemicals in the brain, such as norepinephrine and serotonin, Hullett says, 'CBT reduces the arousal that impacts these chemicals.' This, in effect, may make the body’s natural pain relief response more powerful.

To treat chronic pain, CBT is most often used together with other methods of pain management. These remedies may include medications, physical therapy, weight loss, massage, or in extreme cases, surgery. But among these various methods of pain control, CBT is often one of the most effective.

Of course, there are many other options, and I've listed some of them below, all of which I have utilised at various stages:

- Specialist pain programs
- Counselling
- Acupuncture
- Gentle massage
- Yoga
- Pilates
- Hydrotherapy
- Osteopathy
- Reflexology
- Bowen therapy
- Kinesiology
- Laughter therapy
- Animal therapy
- White laser therapy
- Personal trainer

Be sure to check that all your practitioners are accredited with their relevant associations and have an understanding of chronic pain. You may need a combination of therapies, and different choices at different stages

If you do not feel they are the right support for you, keep looking.

Remember, you are in control of this.

# APPENDIX 4

# RESOURCES AND WEBSITES

## Useful Sites and Articles

Agency for Clinical Innovation
www.aci.health.nsw.gov.au

Australian Pain Management Association
www.painmanagement.org.au

Chronic Pain Australia
www.chronicpainaustralia.org.au

Curable Health
www.curablehealth.com

Dr Carli Axford
www.drcarliaxford.com

*EMDR in the Treatment of Chronic Pain,* Grant M, Threlfo C, Journal of Clinical Psychology, 2002 Dec, 58 (12): 1505-20

JAMA Network, *Reassuring Patients About Low Back Pain* www.jamanetwork.com/journals/jamainternalmedicine/article-abstract/2204030

Mental Health Academy, *Managing Chronic Pain course* www.mentalhealthacademy.com.au/catalogue/courses/managing-chronic-pain

Mindspot Clinic www.mindspot.org.au/

NBCI, Brazilian Journal of Physical Therapy, *Reassurance for patients with non-specific conditions—a user's guide* www.ncbi.nlm.nih.gov/pmc/articles/PMC5537438/

NPS MedicineWise, *Australian Prescriber An Independent Review* www.nps.org.au/australianprescriber

Pain Australia www.painaustralia.org.au

Pain Australia *Chronic Pain Language Guidelines* www.painaustralia.org.au/static/uploads/files/chronic-pain-language-guidelines-wfvxpbiiedsz.pdf

Pure-Li Yoga www.pure-liyoga.com

University of Queensland eSpace, *The Psycho-social Impact of fatal Child Drowning in Queensland and the Availability and Use of Support* www.espace.library.uq.edu.au/view/UQ:341848

Yoga International, *Restorative Yoga for Chronic Pain* www.yogainternational.com/article/view/restorative-yoga-for-chronic-pain

WebMD, *Managing Chronic Pain: A Cognitive-Behavioral Therapy Approach,* Elizabeth Shimer Bowers www.webmd.com/pain-management/features/cognitive-behavioral#1

## Useful Books

*All in My Head,* Paula Kamen, Da Capo Lifelong Books, 2006

*Explain Pain,* David S. Butler and G. Lorimer Moseley. Noigroup Publications, Adelaide, Australia, 2013

*Manage Your Pain, Practical and positive ways of adapting to chronic pain,* Dr Michael Nicholas, Dr Allan Molloy, Lois Tonkin, Lee Beeston. ABC Books, 2011

*Nothing Changes if Nothing Changes. A practical Guide to Choosing the Right Counsellor.* Dawn Spinks, Spinks and Associates Pty Ltd, 2008

*Rewire Your Pain, An evidence-based approach to reducing chronic pain,* Dr Stephanie Davies; Dr Nicolas Cooke, Julia Sutton. WA Specialist Pain Services, 2015

*The Many Parts of You:* Understanding the puzzle of your behaviour, Jan Sky, Balboa Press, Australia, 2012

*What Patients Don't Say if Doctors Don't Ask, The Mindful Patient-Doctor Relationship,* Dr Manon Bollinger,. Influence Publishing Inc, Canada 2014

# ABOUT THE AUTHOR

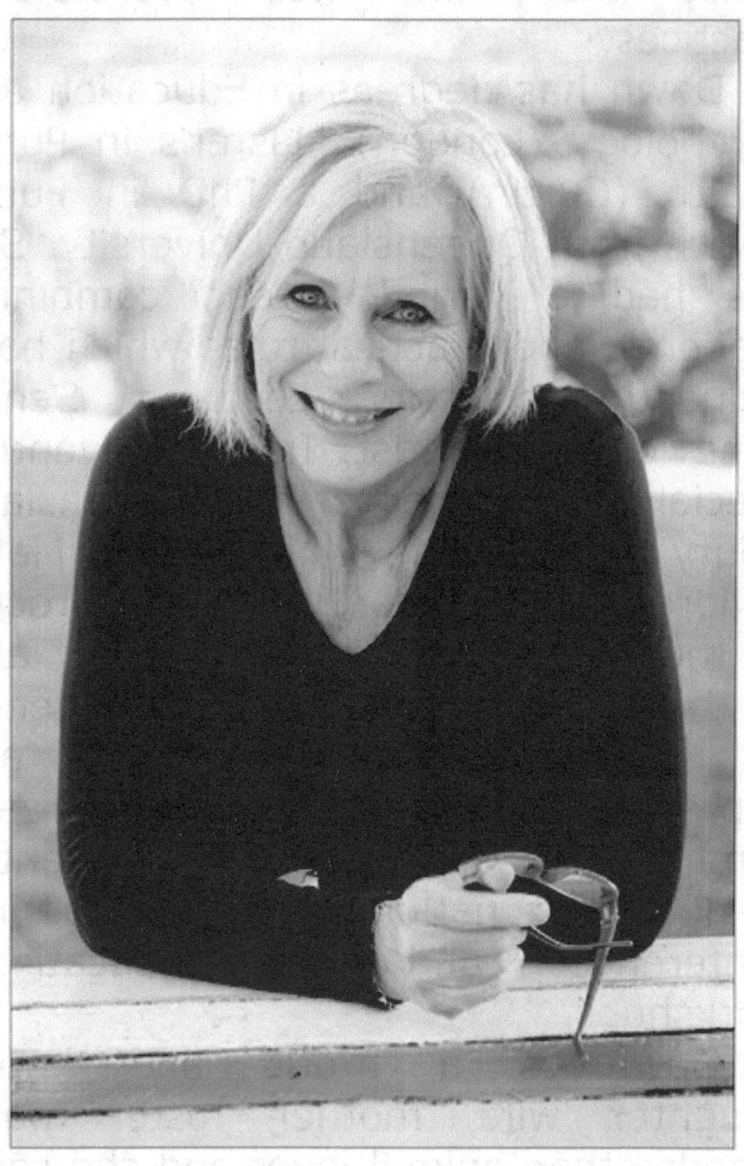

Dawn Macintyre is an experienced clinical counsellor who has worked in her own private practice for nearly three decades and supervises counsellors to assist them in their professional practices.

Dawn has degrees in Education and Psychology (London) Master's in Public Health (Curtin) and a PhD in Public Health from Queensland University. She has had a varied career, combining academic and practical roles which have included University Lecturer, Senior Behavioural Scientist, Injury Prevention specialist, Manager of the Queensland Injury Surveillance Unit at the Mater Children's Hospital, Brisbane, Director of the Safe Communities Centre, also at the Mater Hospital, and Manager of an early intervention anxiety and depression program for hard to reach communities. She has also presented at numerous national and international conferences and runs educational workshops.

Dawn is a proud and happy daughter, wife, mother, foster mum, grandmother, animal lover and she says, hopefully, good friend. She has 4 rescue 'oodles' and 4 alpacas who are a major part of her life, living 'her dream' in the

Northern Rivers, NSW. Dawn and her husband Neil own Highland Retreat, providing a sanctuary amidst the beauty of rolling green hills, for families who may need some respite from life's daily challenges.

Dawn's personal and professional life reflects her passion to make a difference, to speak up when others are silent and to actively provide opportunities for every person to become the best they can be.

Dawn hopes that this book also represents the voice of many, so we can collectively have a better understanding of life with chronic pain and find the support we need to be the best we can be.

# Find out more:

www.drdawnmacintyre.com

www.highlandretreat.com.auwww.oodles offun.com.au

**Facebook:** Dr Dawn Macintrye – Author, Speaker, Facilitator

**Youtube:** Dr Dawn Macintyre

**For more great titles visit**

www.bigskypublishing.com.au

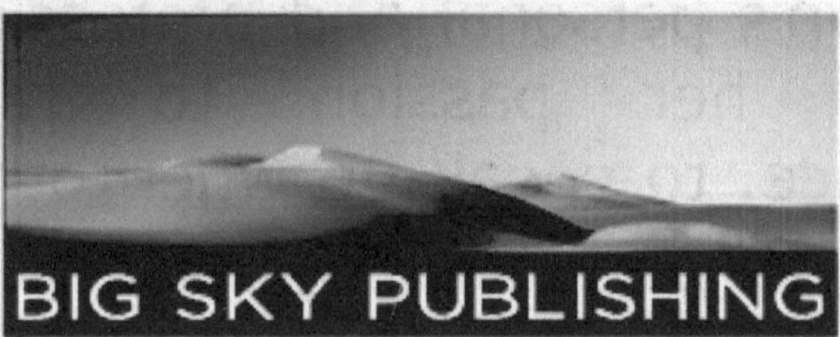

# BACK COVER MATERIAL

**'This book is a clear window into chronic pain. It also contemplates the bright horizon.'**
Elizabeth Carrigan
CEO, Australian Pain Management Association Limited

One in five people live with chronic pain and most feel misunderstood and unsupported. Dr Dawn Macintyre was one of those people. In *Living with Chronic Pain,* Dawn shares her journey from living a full life to a life so diminished, full of pain, shame and exhaustion that she was desperate enough to want to take her own life.

The author's personal story is interwoven with insight into emotions and challenges faced, as well as practical advice for changes and support to help sufferers enjoy life again. Dawn provides a unique perspective as she is both a sufferer of chronic pain and a health practitioner helping people navigate life's challenges.

If you are a health professional, this book offers insight into how to best support your patients and clients living with chronic pain. If you know someone living with chronic pain, reading this book will help you understand and support them. If you are living with chronic pain, this story will bring you courage, joy and most importantly, the knowledge to find your meaningful life again.

www.ingramcontent.com/pod-product-compliance
Lightning Source LLC
LaVergne TN
LVHW030913080826
845145LV00011B/2879

* 9 7 8 0 3 6 9 3 9 1 0 4 9 *